# MY 90 DAY KETO JOURNAL

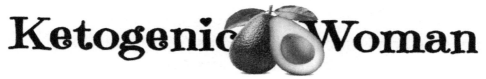

**Ketogenic Woman**

This journal was created by Anita Breeze at
www.ketogenicwoman.com

Join the conversation on Facebook at
https://www.facebook.com/groups/KetogenicWoman

Follow me on Instagram at
http://www.instagram.com/ketogenic.woman

# Ketogenic Woman

# THANK YOU

As a thank you for buying my journal, I am providing you with some helpful resources that can help you along your Keto journey.

Stuck in a plateau?
Learn how the Egg Fast can help at https://ketogenicwoman.com/egg-diet-weight-loss-fast/

Get your free printables at
https://ketogenicwoman.com/egg-fast-printables/

Get your free grocery list at
https://ketogenicwoman.com/getting-started-keto-diet-plan/

And make sure you sign up for my newsletter while you're on the site so you can get delicious recipes delivered straight to your email inbox.

Thank you for buying the My 90 Day Keto Journal!

Now, let's get started!

- Anita

# DAY 1 – STARTING WEIGHT

## Measurements

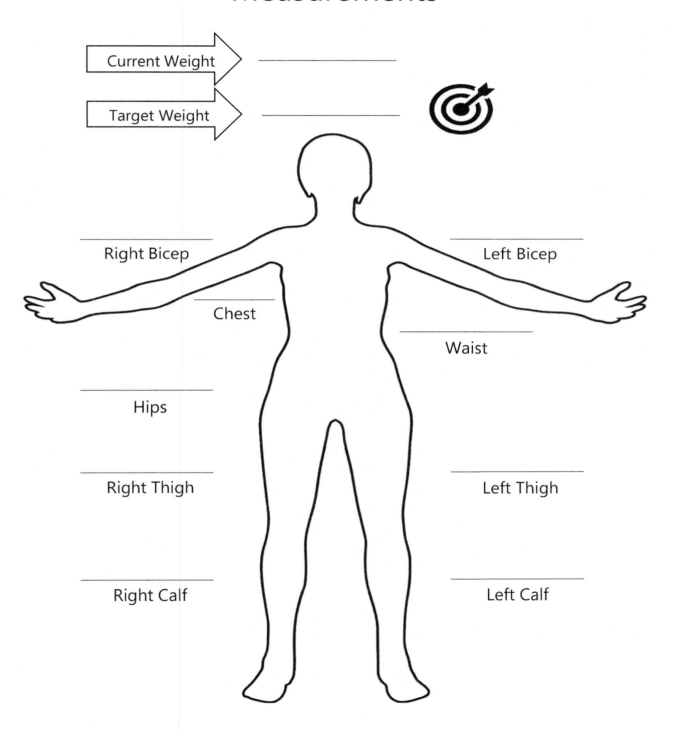

Current Weight ————————————

Target Weight ————————————

Right Bicep

Left Bicep

Chest

Waist

Hips

Right Thigh

Left Thigh

Right Calf

Left Calf

# Questions To Ask Myself

Why am I starting the Keto lifestyle?

_____

_____

_____

_____

What's my end goal?

_____

_____

_____

_____

Do I have a weight loss mindset?

_____

_____

_____

_____

Who can I count on for support?

_____

_____

_____

_____

# DAY 1 - 7

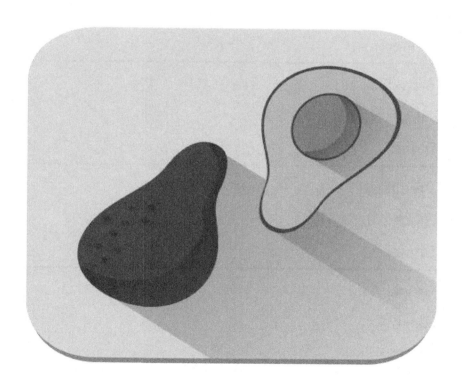

# Meal Planner

| | |
|---|---|
| Day 1 | Breakfast:<br><br>Lunch:<br><br>Dinner: |
| Day 2 | Breakfast:<br><br>Lunch:<br><br>Dinner: |
| Day 3 | Breakfast:<br><br>Lunch:<br><br>Dinner: |
| Day 4 | Breakfast:<br><br>Lunch:<br><br>Dinner: |
| Day 5 | Breakfast:<br><br>Lunch:<br><br>Dinner: |
| Day 6 | Breakfast:<br><br>Lunch:<br><br>Dinner: |
| Day 7 | Breakfast:<br><br>Lunch:<br><br>Dinner: |
| Snacks | |

# Exercise Tracker

| Day 1 |
|---|
| |
| Cardio ◯ |
| Weights ◯ |

| Day 2 |
|---|
| |
| Cardio ◯ |
| Weights ◯ |

| Day 3 |
|---|
| |
| Cardio ◯ |
| Weights ◯ |

| Day 4 |
|---|
| |
| Cardio ◯ |
| Weights ◯ |

| Day 5 |
|---|
| |
| Cardio ◯ |
| Weights ◯ |

| Day 6 |
|---|
| |
| Cardio ◯ |
| Weights ◯ |

| Day 7 |
|---|
| |
| Cardio ◯ |
| Weights ◯ |

| Day | Calories Burned |
|---|---|
| 1 | |
| 2 | |
| 3 | |
| 4 | |
| 5 | |
| 6 | |
| 7 | |

# Day 1    Food Tracker    Date: _____

| ⊕ **Daily Target** | | | | | | |
|---|---|---|---|---|---|---|
| **Breakfast** | Calories | Fat | Protein | Carbs | Fiber | Net Carbs |
| | | | | | | |
| | | | | | | |
| | | | | | | |
| | | | | | | |
| Total: | | | | | | |
| **Lunch** | Calories | Fat | Protein | Carbs | Fiber | Net Carbs |
| | | | | | | |
| | | | | | | |
| | | | | | | |
| | | | | | | |
| Total: | | | | | | |
| **Dinner** | Calories | Fat | Protein | Carbs | Fiber | Net Carbs |
| | | | | | | |
| | | | | | | |
| | | | | | | |
| | | | | | | |
| Total: | | | | | | |
| **Snacks** | Calories | Fat | Protein | Carbs | Fiber | Net Carbs |
| | | | | | | |
| | | | | | | |
| | | | | | | |
| Total: | | | | | | |
| **Daily Total** | | | | | | |

**Ketosis:**   Y/N    Intermittent Fasting: From _____am/pm  -  To_____am/pm

# Day 2    Food Tracker    Date: _____
MON TUE WED THU FRI SAT SUN

| 🎯 **Daily Target** | | | | | | |
|---|---|---|---|---|---|---|
| **Breakfast** | Calories | Fat | Protein | Carbs | Fiber | Net Carbs |
| | | | | | | |
| | | | | | | |
| | | | | | | |
| | | | | | | |
| Total: | | | | | | |
| **Lunch** | Calories | Fat | Protein | Carbs | Fiber | Net Carbs |
| | | | | | | |
| | | | | | | |
| | | | | | | |
| | | | | | | |
| Total: | | | | | | |
| **Dinner** | Calories | Fat | Protein | Carbs | Fiber | Net Carbs |
| | | | | | | |
| | | | | | | |
| | | | | | | |
| | | | | | | |
| Total: | | | | | | |
| **Snacks** | Calories | Fat | Protein | Carbs | Fiber | Net Carbs |
| | | | | | | |
| | | | | | | |
| | | | | | | |
| Total: | | | | | | |
| **Daily Total** | | | | | | |

**Ketosis:**   Y/N      Intermittent Fasting: From _____am/pm  -  To_____am/pm

# Day 3    Food Tracker    Date: _____

| ⊕ **Daily Target** | | | | | | |
|---|---|---|---|---|---|---|
| **Breakfast** | Calories | Fat | Protein | Carbs | Fiber | Net Carbs |
| | | | | | | |
| | | | | | | |
| | | | | | | |
| | | | | | | |
| Total: | | | | | | |
| **Lunch** | Calories | Fat | Protein | Carbs | Fiber | Net Carbs |
| | | | | | | |
| | | | | | | |
| | | | | | | |
| | | | | | | |
| Total: | | | | | | |
| **Dinner** | Calories | Fat | Protein | Carbs | Fiber | Net Carbs |
| | | | | | | |
| | | | | | | |
| | | | | | | |
| | | | | | | |
| Total: | | | | | | |
| **Snacks** | Calories | Fat | Protein | Carbs | Fiber | Net Carbs |
| | | | | | | |
| | | | | | | |
| | | | | | | |
| Total: | | | | | | |
| **Daily Total** | | | | | | |

**Ketosis:**   Y/N    Intermittent Fasting: From _____am/pm  -  To_____am/pm

# Day 4   Food Tracker

Date: _____

| ⊕ Daily Target | | | | | | |
|---|---|---|---|---|---|---|
| **Breakfast** | Calories | Fat | Protein | Carbs | Fiber | Net Carbs |
| | | | | | | |
| | | | | | | |
| | | | | | | |
| Total: | | | | | | |
| **Lunch** | Calories | Fat | Protein | Carbs | Fiber | Net Carbs |
| | | | | | | |
| | | | | | | |
| | | | | | | |
| Total: | | | | | | |
| **Dinner** | Calories | Fat | Protein | Carbs | Fiber | Net Carbs |
| | | | | | | |
| | | | | | | |
| | | | | | | |
| Total: | | | | | | |
| **Snacks** | Calories | Fat | Protein | Carbs | Fiber | Net Carbs |
| | | | | | | |
| | | | | | | |
| | | | | | | |
| Total: | | | | | | |
| **Daily Total** | | | | | | |

**Ketosis:**   Y/N     Intermittent Fasting: From _____am/pm - To_____am/pm

# Day 5     Food Tracker

Date: _____
MON TUE WED THU FRI SAT SUN

| 🎯 Daily Target | | | | | | |
|---|---|---|---|---|---|---|
| **Breakfast** | Calories | Fat | Protein | Carbs | Fiber | Net Carbs |
| | | | | | | |
| | | | | | | |
| | | | | | | |
| | | | | | | |
| Total: | | | | | | |
| **Lunch** | Calories | Fat | Protein | Carbs | Fiber | Net Carbs |
| | | | | | | |
| | | | | | | |
| | | | | | | |
| | | | | | | |
| Total: | | | | | | |
| **Dinner** | Calories | Fat | Protein | Carbs | Fiber | Net Carbs |
| | | | | | | |
| | | | | | | |
| | | | | | | |
| | | | | | | |
| Total: | | | | | | |
| **Snacks** | Calories | Fat | Protein | Carbs | Fiber | Net Carbs |
| | | | | | | |
| | | | | | | |
| | | | | | | |
| Total: | | | | | | |
| **Daily Total** | | | | | | |

**Ketosis:**   Y/N    Intermittent Fasting: From _____am/pm  - To_____am/pm

# Day 6     Food Tracker     Date: _____

MON TUE WED THU FRI SAT SUN

| 🎯 **Daily Target** | | | | | | |
|---|---|---|---|---|---|---|
| **Breakfast** | Calories | Fat | Protein | Carbs | Fiber | Net Carbs |
| | | | | | | |
| | | | | | | |
| | | | | | | |
| | | | | | | |
| Total: | | | | | | |
| **Lunch** | Calories | Fat | Protein | Carbs | Fiber | Net Carbs |
| | | | | | | |
| | | | | | | |
| | | | | | | |
| | | | | | | |
| Total: | | | | | | |
| **Dinner** | Calories | Fat | Protein | Carbs | Fiber | Net Carbs |
| | | | | | | |
| | | | | | | |
| | | | | | | |
| | | | | | | |
| Total: | | | | | | |
| **Snacks** | Calories | Fat | Protein | Carbs | Fiber | Net Carbs |
| | | | | | | |
| | | | | | | |
| | | | | | | |
| Total: | | | | | | |
| **Daily Total** | | | | | | |

**Ketosis:**   Y/N     Intermittent Fasting: From _____am/pm  -  To_____am/pm

# Day 7    Food Tracker

Date: _____

| 🎯 Daily Target | | | | | | |
|---|---|---|---|---|---|---|
| **Breakfast** | Calories | Fat | Protein | Carbs | Fiber | Net Carbs |
| | | | | | | |
| | | | | | | |
| | | | | | | |
| | | | | | | |
| Total: | | | | | | |
| **Lunch** | Calories | Fat | Protein | Carbs | Fiber | Net Carbs |
| | | | | | | |
| | | | | | | |
| | | | | | | |
| | | | | | | |
| Total: | | | | | | |
| **Dinner** | Calories | Fat | Protein | Carbs | Fiber | Net Carbs |
| | | | | | | |
| | | | | | | |
| | | | | | | |
| | | | | | | |
| Total: | | | | | | |
| **Snacks** | Calories | Fat | Protein | Carbs | Fiber | Net Carbs |
| | | | | | | |
| | | | | | | |
| | | | | | | |
| Total: | | | | | | |
| **Daily Total** | | | | | | |

**Ketosis:**   Y/N    Intermittent Fasting: From _____am/pm - To_____am/pm

# NOTES

# DAY 8 – WEIGHT
## Measurements

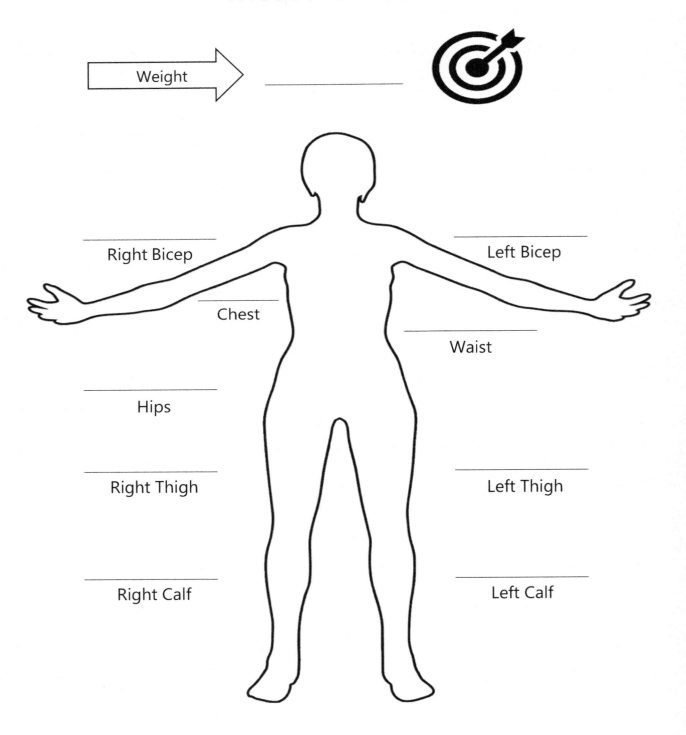

Weight _____

Right Bicep _____

Left Bicep _____

Chest _____

Waist _____

Hips _____

Right Thigh _____

Left Thigh _____

Right Calf _____

Left Calf _____

# Questions To Ask Yourself

Am I happy with my results after the last 7 days?

_____

_____

_____

_____

What was my biggest win?

_____

_____

_____

What adjustments should I make?

_____

_____

_____

How does my body feel?

_____

_____

_____

# DAY 8 - 14

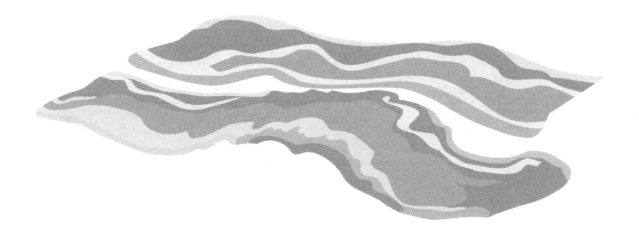

# Meal Planner

Day 8 - 14

| | |
|---|---|
| **Day 1** | Breakfast:<br>Lunch:<br>Dinner: |
| **Day 2** | Breakfast:<br>Lunch:<br>Dinner: |
| **Day 3** | Breakfast:<br>Lunch:<br>Dinner: |
| **Day 4** | Breakfast:<br>Lunch:<br>Dinner: |
| **Day 5** | Breakfast:<br>Lunch:<br>Dinner: |
| **Day 6** | Breakfast:<br>Lunch:<br>Dinner: |
| **Day 7** | Breakfast:<br>Lunch:<br>Dinner: |
| **Snacks** | |

# Exercise Tracker

Day 8 - 14

| Day 1 | Day 2 | Day 3 |
|---|---|---|
| | | |

Cardio ◯   Cardio ◯   Cardio ◯
Weights ◯   Weights ◯   Weights ◯

| Day 4 | Day 5 | Day 6 |
|---|---|---|
| | | |

Cardio ◯   Cardio ◯   Cardio ◯
Weights ◯   Weights ◯   Weights ◯

| Day 7 |
|---|
| |

Cardio ◯
Weights ◯

| Day | Calories Burned |
|---|---|
| 1 | |
| 2 | |
| 3 | |
| 4 | |
| 5 | |
| 6 | |
| 7 | |

# Day 8     Food Tracker    Date: _____

| 🎯 Daily Target | | | | | | |
|---|---|---|---|---|---|---|
| **Breakfast** | Calories | Fat | Protein | Carbs | Fiber | Net Carbs |
| | | | | | | |
| | | | | | | |
| | | | | | | |
| | | | | | | |
| Total: | | | | | | |
| **Lunch** | Calories | Fat | Protein | Carbs | Fiber | Net Carbs |
| | | | | | | |
| | | | | | | |
| | | | | | | |
| | | | | | | |
| Total: | | | | | | |
| **Dinner** | Calories | Fat | Protein | Carbs | Fiber | Net Carbs |
| | | | | | | |
| | | | | | | |
| | | | | | | |
| | | | | | | |
| Total: | | | | | | |
| **Snacks** | Calories | Fat | Protein | Carbs | Fiber | Net Carbs |
| | | | | | | |
| | | | | | | |
| | | | | | | |
| Total: | | | | | | |
| **Daily Total** | | | | | | |

**Ketosis:**   Y/N    Intermittent Fasting: From _____am/pm - To_____am/pm

# Day 9    Food Tracker

Date: _____
MON TUE WED THU FRI SAT SUN

| 🎯 Daily Target | | | | | | |
|---|---|---|---|---|---|---|
| **Breakfast** | Calories | Fat | Protein | Carbs | Fiber | Net Carbs |
| | | | | | | |
| | | | | | | |
| | | | | | | |
| | | | | | | |
| Total: | | | | | | |
| **Lunch** | Calories | Fat | Protein | Carbs | Fiber | Net Carbs |
| | | | | | | |
| | | | | | | |
| | | | | | | |
| | | | | | | |
| Total: | | | | | | |
| **Dinner** | Calories | Fat | Protein | Carbs | Fiber | Net Carbs |
| | | | | | | |
| | | | | | | |
| | | | | | | |
| | | | | | | |
| Total: | | | | | | |
| **Snacks** | Calories | Fat | Protein | Carbs | Fiber | Net Carbs |
| | | | | | | |
| | | | | | | |
| | | | | | | |
| Total: | | | | | | |
| **Daily Total** | | | | | | |

**Ketosis:**   Y/N    Intermittent Fasting: From _____am/pm - To_____am/pm

# Day 10    Food Tracker

Date: _____

| 🎯 Daily Target | | | | | | |
|---|---|---|---|---|---|---|
| **Breakfast** | Calories | Fat | Protein | Carbs | Fiber | Net Carbs |
| | | | | | | |
| | | | | | | |
| | | | | | | |
| | | | | | | |
| Total: | | | | | | |
| **Lunch** | Calories | Fat | Protein | Carbs | Fiber | Net Carbs |
| | | | | | | |
| | | | | | | |
| | | | | | | |
| | | | | | | |
| Total: | | | | | | |
| **Dinner** | Calories | Fat | Protein | Carbs | Fiber | Net Carbs |
| | | | | | | |
| | | | | | | |
| | | | | | | |
| | | | | | | |
| Total: | | | | | | |
| **Snacks** | Calories | Fat | Protein | Carbs | Fiber | Net Carbs |
| | | | | | | |
| | | | | | | |
| | | | | | | |
| Total: | | | | | | |
| **Daily Total** | | | | | | |

**Ketosis:**   Y/N    Intermittent Fasting: From _____am/pm - To_____am/pm

# Day 11    Food Tracker

Date: _____

MON TUE WED THU FRI SAT SUN

| 🎯 Daily Target | | | | | | |
|---|---|---|---|---|---|---|
| **Breakfast** | Calories | Fat | Protein | Carbs | Fiber | Net Carbs |
| | | | | | | |
| | | | | | | |
| | | | | | | |
| | | | | | | |
| Total: | | | | | | |
| **Lunch** | Calories | Fat | Protein | Carbs | Fiber | Net Carbs |
| | | | | | | |
| | | | | | | |
| | | | | | | |
| | | | | | | |
| Total: | | | | | | |
| **Dinner** | Calories | Fat | Protein | Carbs | Fiber | Net Carbs |
| | | | | | | |
| | | | | | | |
| | | | | | | |
| | | | | | | |
| Total: | | | | | | |
| **Snacks** | Calories | Fat | Protein | Carbs | Fiber | Net Carbs |
| | | | | | | |
| | | | | | | |
| | | | | | | |
| Total: | | | | | | |
| **Daily Total** | | | | | | |

**Ketosis:**   Y/N      Intermittent Fasting: From _____am/pm - To_____am/pm

# Day 12    Food Tracker

Date: _____

MON TUE WED THU FRI SAT SUN

| 🎯 **Daily Target** | | | | | | |
|---|---|---|---|---|---|---|
| **Breakfast** | Calories | Fat | Protein | Carbs | Fiber | Net Carbs |
| | | | | | | |
| | | | | | | |
| | | | | | | |
| | | | | | | |
| Total: | | | | | | |
| **Lunch** | Calories | Fat | Protein | Carbs | Fiber | Net Carbs |
| | | | | | | |
| | | | | | | |
| | | | | | | |
| | | | | | | |
| Total: | | | | | | |
| **Dinner** | Calories | Fat | Protein | Carbs | Fiber | Net Carbs |
| | | | | | | |
| | | | | | | |
| | | | | | | |
| | | | | | | |
| Total: | | | | | | |
| **Snacks** | Calories | Fat | Protein | Carbs | Fiber | Net Carbs |
| | | | | | | |
| | | | | | | |
| | | | | | | |
| Total: | | | | | | |
| **Daily Total** | | | | | | |

**Ketosis:** Y/N    Intermittent Fasting: From _____am/pm - To_____am/pm

# Day 13  Food Tracker

Date: _____

| 🎯 Daily Target | | | | | | |
|---|---|---|---|---|---|---|
| **Breakfast** | Calories | Fat | Protein | Carbs | Fiber | Net Carbs |
| | | | | | | |
| | | | | | | |
| | | | | | | |
| | | | | | | |
| Total: | | | | | | |
| **Lunch** | Calories | Fat | Protein | Carbs | Fiber | Net Carbs |
| | | | | | | |
| | | | | | | |
| | | | | | | |
| | | | | | | |
| Total: | | | | | | |
| **Dinner** | Calories | Fat | Protein | Carbs | Fiber | Net Carbs |
| | | | | | | |
| | | | | | | |
| | | | | | | |
| | | | | | | |
| Total: | | | | | | |
| **Snacks** | Calories | Fat | Protein | Carbs | Fiber | Net Carbs |
| | | | | | | |
| | | | | | | |
| | | | | | | |
| Total: | | | | | | |
| **Daily Total** | | | | | | |

**Ketosis:**   Y/N     Intermittent Fasting: From _____am/pm  -  To_____am/pm

# Day 14    Food Tracker    Date: _____

| 🎯 Daily Target | | | | | | |
|---|---|---|---|---|---|---|
| **Breakfast** | Calories | Fat | Protein | Carbs | Fiber | Net Carbs |
| | | | | | | |
| | | | | | | |
| | | | | | | |
| | | | | | | |
| Total: | | | | | | |
| **Lunch** | Calories | Fat | Protein | Carbs | Fiber | Net Carbs |
| | | | | | | |
| | | | | | | |
| | | | | | | |
| | | | | | | |
| Total: | | | | | | |
| **Dinner** | Calories | Fat | Protein | Carbs | Fiber | Net Carbs |
| | | | | | | |
| | | | | | | |
| | | | | | | |
| | | | | | | |
| Total: | | | | | | |
| **Snacks** | Calories | Fat | Protein | Carbs | Fiber | Net Carbs |
| | | | | | | |
| | | | | | | |
| Total: | | | | | | |
| **Daily Total** | | | | | | |

**Ketosis:**   Y/N    Intermittent Fasting: From _____am/pm - To_____am/pm

# NOTES

# DAY 15 – WEIGHT

## Measurements

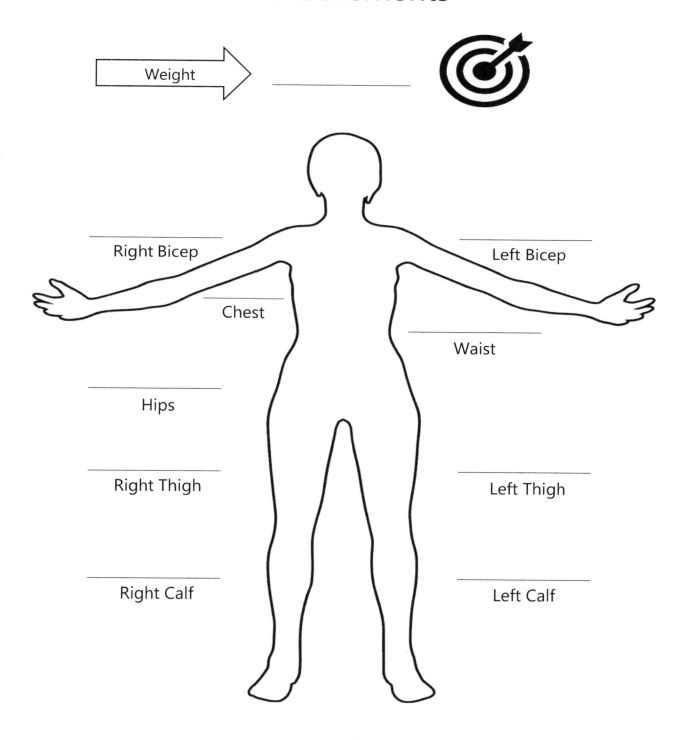

# Questions To Ask Yourself

Am I happy with my results after the last 7 days?

_____

_____

_____

_____

What was my biggest win?

_____

_____

_____

_____

What adjustments should I make?

_____

_____

_____

_____

How does my body feel?

_____

_____

_____

_____

# DAY 15 - 21

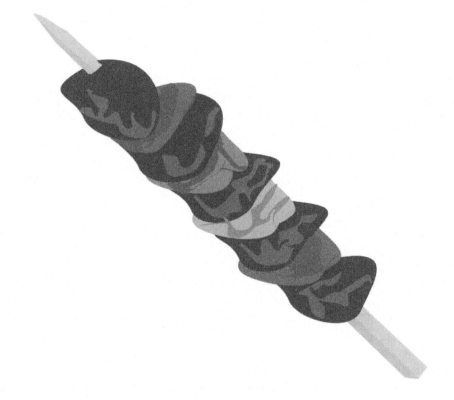

# Meal Planner

Day 15 - 21

| | |
|---|---|
| Day 1 | Breakfast:<br><br>Lunch:<br><br>Dinner: |
| Day 2 | Breakfast:<br><br>Lunch:<br><br>Dinner: |
| Day 3 | Breakfast:<br><br>Lunch:<br><br>Dinner: |
| Day 4 | Breakfast:<br><br>Lunch:<br><br>Dinner: |
| Day 5 | Breakfast:<br><br>Lunch:<br><br>Dinner: |
| Day 6 | Breakfast:<br><br>Lunch:<br><br>Dinner: |
| Day 7 | Breakfast:<br><br>Lunch:<br><br>Dinner: |
| Snacks | |

# Exercise Tracker

Day 15 - 21

| Day 1 |
|---|
| |
| Cardio ◯ |
| Weights ◯ |

| Day 2 |
|---|
| |
| Cardio ◯ |
| Weights ◯ |

| Day 3 |
|---|
| |
| Cardio ◯ |
| Weights ◯ |

| Day 4 |
|---|
| |
| Cardio ◯ |
| Weights ◯ |

| Day 5 |
|---|
| |
| Cardio ◯ |
| Weights ◯ |

| Day 6 |
|---|
| |
| Cardio ◯ |
| Weights ◯ |

| Day 7 |
|---|
| |
| Cardio ◯ |
| Weights ◯ |

| Day | Calories Burned |
|---|---|
| 1 | |
| 2 | |
| 3 | |
| 4 | |
| 5 | |
| 6 | |
| 7 | |

# Day 15      Food Tracker      Date: _____

| ⊕ Daily Target | | | | | | |
|---|---|---|---|---|---|---|
| **Breakfast** | Calories | Fat | Protein | Carbs | Fiber | Net Carbs |
| | | | | | | |
| | | | | | | |
| | | | | | | |
| | | | | | | |
| Total: | | | | | | |
| **Lunch** | Calories | Fat | Protein | Carbs | Fiber | Net Carbs |
| | | | | | | |
| | | | | | | |
| | | | | | | |
| | | | | | | |
| Total: | | | | | | |
| **Dinner** | Calories | Fat | Protein | Carbs | Fiber | Net Carbs |
| | | | | | | |
| | | | | | | |
| | | | | | | |
| | | | | | | |
| Total: | | | | | | |
| **Snacks** | Calories | Fat | Protein | Carbs | Fiber | Net Carbs |
| | | | | | | |
| | | | | | | |
| | | | | | | |
| Total: | | | | | | |
| **Daily Total** | | | | | | |

**Ketosis:**   Y/N      Intermittent Fasting: From _____am/pm - To_____am/pm

# Day 16    Food Tracker

Date: _____

| 🎯 Daily Target | | | | | | |
|---|---|---|---|---|---|---|
| **Breakfast** | Calories | Fat | Protein | Carbs | Fiber | Net Carbs |
| | | | | | | |
| | | | | | | |
| | | | | | | |
| Total: | | | | | | |
| **Lunch** | Calories | Fat | Protein | Carbs | Fiber | Net Carbs |
| | | | | | | |
| | | | | | | |
| | | | | | | |
| Total: | | | | | | |
| **Dinner** | Calories | Fat | Protein | Carbs | Fiber | Net Carbs |
| | | | | | | |
| | | | | | | |
| | | | | | | |
| Total: | | | | | | |
| **Snacks** | Calories | Fat | Protein | Carbs | Fiber | Net Carbs |
| | | | | | | |
| | | | | | | |
| Total: | | | | | | |
| **Daily Total** | | | | | | |

**Ketosis:**   Y/N     Intermittent Fasting: From _____am/pm - To_____am/pm

# Day 17　Food Tracker

| 🎯 Daily Target | | | | | | |
|---|---|---|---|---|---|---|

| **Breakfast** | Calories | Fat | Protein | Carbs | Fiber | Net Carbs |
|---|---|---|---|---|---|---|
| | | | | | | |
| | | | | | | |
| | | | | | | |
| Total: | | | | | | |

| **Lunch** | Calories | Fat | Protein | Carbs | Fiber | Net Carbs |
|---|---|---|---|---|---|---|
| | | | | | | |
| | | | | | | |
| | | | | | | |
| Total: | | | | | | |

| **Dinner** | Calories | Fat | Protein | Carbs | Fiber | Net Carbs |
|---|---|---|---|---|---|---|
| | | | | | | |
| | | | | | | |
| | | | | | | |
| | | | | | | |
| Total: | | | | | | |

| **Snacks** | Calories | Fat | Protein | Carbs | Fiber | Net Carbs |
|---|---|---|---|---|---|---|
| | | | | | | |
| | | | | | | |
| | | | | | | |
| Total: | | | | | | |

| **Daily Total** | | | | | | |
|---|---|---|---|---|---|---|

**Ketosis:**　Y/N　Intermittent Fasting: From _____am/pm - To_____am/pm

# Day 18    Food Tracker    Date: _____

MON TUE WED THU FRI SAT SUN

| 🎯 **Daily Target** | | | | | | |
|---|---|---|---|---|---|---|
| **Breakfast** | Calories | Fat | Protein | Carbs | Fiber | Net Carbs |
| | | | | | | |
| | | | | | | |
| | | | | | | |
| | | | | | | |
| Total: | | | | | | |
| **Lunch** | Calories | Fat | Protein | Carbs | Fiber | Net Carbs |
| | | | | | | |
| | | | | | | |
| | | | | | | |
| | | | | | | |
| Total: | | | | | | |
| **Dinner** | Calories | Fat | Protein | Carbs | Fiber | Net Carbs |
| | | | | | | |
| | | | | | | |
| | | | | | | |
| | | | | | | |
| Total: | | | | | | |
| **Snacks** | Calories | Fat | Protein | Carbs | Fiber | Net Carbs |
| | | | | | | |
| | | | | | | |
| | | | | | | |
| Total: | | | | | | |
| **Daily Total** | | | | | | |

**Ketosis:** Y/N    Intermittent Fasting: From _____am/pm - To_____am/pm

# Day 19    Food Tracker

Date: _____

MON TUE WED THU FRI SAT SUN

| 🎯 Daily Target | | | | | | |
|---|---|---|---|---|---|---|
| **Breakfast** | Calories | Fat | Protein | Carbs | Fiber | Net Carbs |
| | | | | | | |
| | | | | | | |
| | | | | | | |
| | | | | | | |
| Total: | | | | | | |
| **Lunch** | Calories | Fat | Protein | Carbs | Fiber | Net Carbs |
| | | | | | | |
| | | | | | | |
| | | | | | | |
| | | | | | | |
| Total: | | | | | | |
| **Dinner** | Calories | Fat | Protein | Carbs | Fiber | Net Carbs |
| | | | | | | |
| | | | | | | |
| | | | | | | |
| | | | | | | |
| Total: | | | | | | |
| **Snacks** | Calories | Fat | Protein | Carbs | Fiber | Net Carbs |
| | | | | | | |
| | | | | | | |
| | | | | | | |
| Total: | | | | | | |
| **Daily Total** | | | | | | |

**Ketosis:**   Y/N    Intermittent Fasting: From _____am/pm - To_____am/pm

# Day 20     Food Tracker     Date: _____

| ⊕ Daily Target | | | | | | |
|---|---|---|---|---|---|---|
| **Breakfast** | Calories | Fat | Protein | Carbs | Fiber | Net Carbs |
| | | | | | | |
| | | | | | | |
| | | | | | | |
| | | | | | | |
| Total: | | | | | | |
| **Lunch** | Calories | Fat | Protein | Carbs | Fiber | Net Carbs |
| | | | | | | |
| | | | | | | |
| | | | | | | |
| | | | | | | |
| Total: | | | | | | |
| **Dinner** | Calories | Fat | Protein | Carbs | Fiber | Net Carbs |
| | | | | | | |
| | | | | | | |
| | | | | | | |
| | | | | | | |
| Total: | | | | | | |
| **Snacks** | Calories | Fat | Protein | Carbs | Fiber | Net Carbs |
| | | | | | | |
| | | | | | | |
| | | | | | | |
| Total: | | | | | | |
| **Daily Total** | | | | | | |

**Ketosis:**   Y/N     Intermittent Fasting: From _____am/pm - To_____am/pm

# Day 21    Food Tracker

| 🎯 Daily Target | | | | | | |
|---|---|---|---|---|---|---|
| **Breakfast** | Calories | Fat | Protein | Carbs | Fiber | Net Carbs |
| | | | | | | |
| | | | | | | |
| | | | | | | |
| | | | | | | |
| Total: | | | | | | |
| **Lunch** | Calories | Fat | Protein | Carbs | Fiber | Net Carbs |
| | | | | | | |
| | | | | | | |
| | | | | | | |
| | | | | | | |
| Total: | | | | | | |
| **Dinner** | Calories | Fat | Protein | Carbs | Fiber | Net Carbs |
| | | | | | | |
| | | | | | | |
| | | | | | | |
| | | | | | | |
| Total: | | | | | | |
| **Snacks** | Calories | Fat | Protein | Carbs | Fiber | Net Carbs |
| | | | | | | |
| | | | | | | |
| | | | | | | |
| Total: | | | | | | |
| **Daily Total** | | | | | | |

**Ketosis:**    Y/N    Intermittent Fasting: From _____am/pm - To_____am/pm

# NOTES

# DAY 22 – WEIGHT

## Measurements

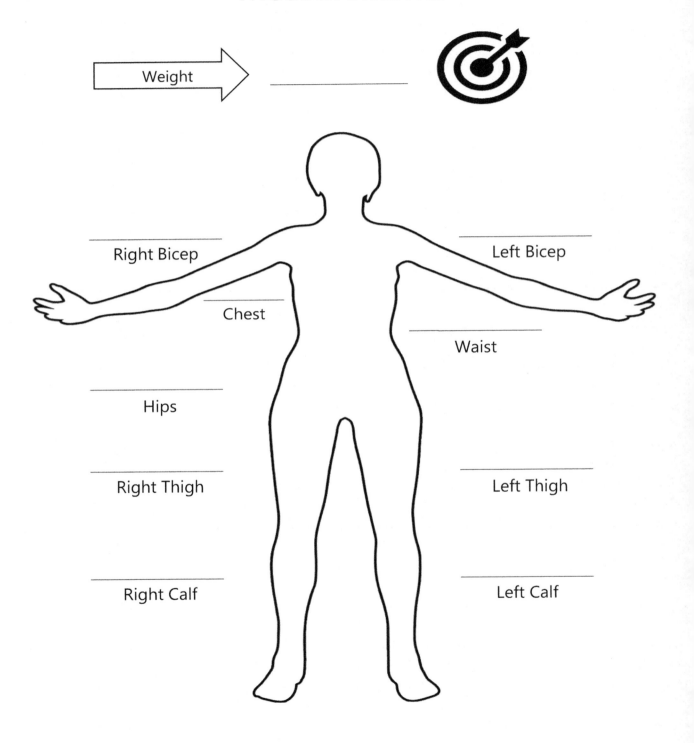

Weight _____

Right Bicep

Left Bicep

Chest

Waist

Hips

Right Thigh

Left Thigh

Right Calf

Left Calf

# Questions To Ask Yourself

Am I happy with my results after the last 7 days?

_____

_____

_____

_____

What was my biggest win?

_____

_____

_____

_____

What adjustments should I make?

_____

_____

_____

_____

How does my body feel?

_____

_____

_____

_____

# DAY 22 - 28

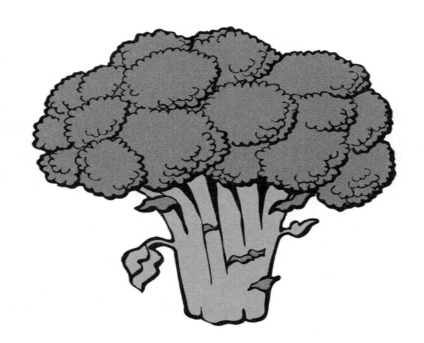

# Meal Planner

Day 22 - 28

| | |
|---|---|
| **Day 1** | Breakfast:<br>Lunch:<br>Dinner: |
| **Day 2** | Breakfast:<br>Lunch:<br>Dinner: |
| **Day 3** | Breakfast:<br>Lunch:<br>Dinner: |
| **Day 4** | Breakfast:<br>Lunch:<br>Dinner: |
| **Day 5** | Breakfast:<br>Lunch:<br>Dinner: |
| **Day 6** | Breakfast:<br>Lunch:<br>Dinner: |
| **Day 7** | Breakfast:<br>Lunch:<br>Dinner: |
| **Snacks** | |

# Exercise Tracker

| Day 1 |
|---|
| |
| Cardio ◯ |
| Weights ◯ |

| Day 2 |
|---|
| |
| Cardio ◯ |
| Weights ◯ |

| Day 3 |
|---|
| |
| Cardio ◯ |
| Weights ◯ |

| Day 4 |
|---|
| |
| Cardio ◯ |
| Weights ◯ |

| Day 5 |
|---|
| |
| Cardio ◯ |
| Weights ◯ |

| Day 6 |
|---|
| |
| Cardio ◯ |
| Weights ◯ |

| Day 7 |
|---|
| |
| Cardio ◯ |
| Weights ◯ |

| Day | Calories Burned |
|---|---|
| 1 | |
| 2 | |
| 3 | |
| 4 | |
| 5 | |
| 6 | |
| 7 | |

# Day 22    Food Tracker    Date: _____
MON TUE WED THU FRI SAT SUN

| ⊕ Daily Target | | | | | | |
|---|---|---|---|---|---|---|
| **Breakfast** | Calories | Fat | Protein | Carbs | Fiber | Net Carbs |
| | | | | | | |
| | | | | | | |
| | | | | | | |
| | | | | | | |
| Total: | | | | | | |
| **Lunch** | Calories | Fat | Protein | Carbs | Fiber | Net Carbs |
| | | | | | | |
| | | | | | | |
| | | | | | | |
| | | | | | | |
| Total: | | | | | | |
| **Dinner** | Calories | Fat | Protein | Carbs | Fiber | Net Carbs |
| | | | | | | |
| | | | | | | |
| | | | | | | |
| | | | | | | |
| Total: | | | | | | |
| **Snacks** | Calories | Fat | Protein | Carbs | Fiber | Net Carbs |
| | | | | | | |
| | | | | | | |
| | | | | | | |
| Total: | | | | | | |
| **Daily Total** | | | | | | |

**Ketosis:**   Y/N      Intermittent Fasting: From _____am/pm - To_____am/pm

# Day 23    Food Tracker    Date: _____

| 🎯 Daily Target | | | | | | |
|---|---|---|---|---|---|---|
| **Breakfast** | Calories | Fat | Protein | Carbs | Fiber | Net Carbs |
| | | | | | | |
| | | | | | | |
| | | | | | | |
| Total: | | | | | | |
| **Lunch** | Calories | Fat | Protein | Carbs | Fiber | Net Carbs |
| | | | | | | |
| | | | | | | |
| | | | | | | |
| Total: | | | | | | |
| **Dinner** | Calories | Fat | Protein | Carbs | Fiber | Net Carbs |
| | | | | | | |
| | | | | | | |
| | | | | | | |
| Total: | | | | | | |
| **Snacks** | Calories | Fat | Protein | Carbs | Fiber | Net Carbs |
| | | | | | | |
| | | | | | | |
| | | | | | | |
| Total: | | | | | | |
| **Daily Total** | | | | | | |

**Ketosis:**   Y/N    Intermittent Fasting: From ____am/pm - To____am/pm

# Day 24    Food Tracker    Date: _____

| 🎯 **Daily Target** | | | | | | |
|---|---|---|---|---|---|---|
| **Breakfast** | Calories | Fat | Protein | Carbs | Fiber | Net Carbs |
| | | | | | | |
| | | | | | | |
| | | | | | | |
| | | | | | | |
| Total: | | | | | | |
| **Lunch** | Calories | Fat | Protein | Carbs | Fiber | Net Carbs |
| | | | | | | |
| | | | | | | |
| | | | | | | |
| | | | | | | |
| Total: | | | | | | |
| **Dinner** | Calories | Fat | Protein | Carbs | Fiber | Net Carbs |
| | | | | | | |
| | | | | | | |
| | | | | | | |
| | | | | | | |
| Total: | | | | | | |
| **Snacks** | Calories | Fat | Protein | Carbs | Fiber | Net Carbs |
| | | | | | | |
| | | | | | | |
| | | | | | | |
| Total: | | | | | | |
| **Daily Total** | | | | | | |

**Ketosis:**   Y/N     Intermittent Fasting: From ____am/pm - To____am/pm

# Day 25    Food Tracker

Date: _____
MON TUE WED THU FRI SAT SUN

| 🎯 Daily Target | | | | | | |
|---|---|---|---|---|---|---|
| **Breakfast** | Calories | Fat | Protein | Carbs | Fiber | Net Carbs |
| | | | | | | |
| | | | | | | |
| | | | | | | |
| | | | | | | |
| Total: | | | | | | |
| **Lunch** | Calories | Fat | Protein | Carbs | Fiber | Net Carbs |
| | | | | | | |
| | | | | | | |
| | | | | | | |
| | | | | | | |
| Total: | | | | | | |
| **Dinner** | Calories | Fat | Protein | Carbs | Fiber | Net Carbs |
| | | | | | | |
| | | | | | | |
| | | | | | | |
| | | | | | | |
| Total: | | | | | | |
| **Snacks** | Calories | Fat | Protein | Carbs | Fiber | Net Carbs |
| | | | | | | |
| | | | | | | |
| | | | | | | |
| Total: | | | | | | |
| **Daily Total** | | | | | | |

**Ketosis:**   Y/N    Intermittent Fasting: From ____am/pm - To____am/pm

# Day 26     Food Tracker

Date: _____

| ⊕ Daily Target | | | | | | |
|---|---|---|---|---|---|---|
| **Breakfast** | Calories | Fat | Protein | Carbs | Fiber | Net Carbs |
| | | | | | | |
| | | | | | | |
| | | | | | | |
| | | | | | | |
| Total: | | | | | | |
| **Lunch** | Calories | Fat | Protein | Carbs | Fiber | Net Carbs |
| | | | | | | |
| | | | | | | |
| | | | | | | |
| | | | | | | |
| Total: | | | | | | |
| **Dinner** | Calories | Fat | Protein | Carbs | Fiber | Net Carbs |
| | | | | | | |
| | | | | | | |
| | | | | | | |
| | | | | | | |
| Total: | | | | | | |
| **Snacks** | Calories | Fat | Protein | Carbs | Fiber | Net Carbs |
| | | | | | | |
| | | | | | | |
| | | | | | | |
| Total: | | | | | | |
| **Daily Total** | | | | | | |

**Ketosis:**   Y/N     Intermittent Fasting: From _____am/pm  -  To_____am/pm

# Day 27    Food Tracker

Date: _____

| 🎯 Daily Target | | | | | | |
|---|---|---|---|---|---|---|
| **Breakfast** | Calories | Fat | Protein | Carbs | Fiber | Net Carbs |
| | | | | | | |
| | | | | | | |
| | | | | | | |
| | | | | | | |
| Total: | | | | | | |
| **Lunch** | Calories | Fat | Protein | Carbs | Fiber | Net Carbs |
| | | | | | | |
| | | | | | | |
| | | | | | | |
| | | | | | | |
| Total: | | | | | | |
| **Dinner** | Calories | Fat | Protein | Carbs | Fiber | Net Carbs |
| | | | | | | |
| | | | | | | |
| | | | | | | |
| | | | | | | |
| Total: | | | | | | |
| **Snacks** | Calories | Fat | Protein | Carbs | Fiber | Net Carbs |
| | | | | | | |
| | | | | | | |
| | | | | | | |
| Total: | | | | | | |
| **Daily Total** | | | | | | |

**Ketosis:**   Y/N    Intermittent Fasting: From _____am/pm - To_____am/pm

# Day 28    Food Tracker

| 🎯 Daily Target | | | | | | |
|---|---|---|---|---|---|---|
| **Breakfast** | Calories | Fat | Protein | Carbs | Fiber | Net Carbs |
| | | | | | | |
| | | | | | | |
| | | | | | | |
| | | | | | | |
| Total: | | | | | | |
| **Lunch** | Calories | Fat | Protein | Carbs | Fiber | Net Carbs |
| | | | | | | |
| | | | | | | |
| | | | | | | |
| | | | | | | |
| Total: | | | | | | |
| **Dinner** | Calories | Fat | Protein | Carbs | Fiber | Net Carbs |
| | | | | | | |
| | | | | | | |
| | | | | | | |
| | | | | | | |
| Total: | | | | | | |
| **Snacks** | Calories | Fat | Protein | Carbs | Fiber | Net Carbs |
| | | | | | | |
| | | | | | | |
| | | | | | | |
| Total: | | | | | | |
| **Daily Total** | | | | | | |

**Ketosis:**   Y/N    Intermittent Fasting: From ____am/pm - To____am/pm

# NOTES

# DAY 29 – WEIGHT

## Measurements

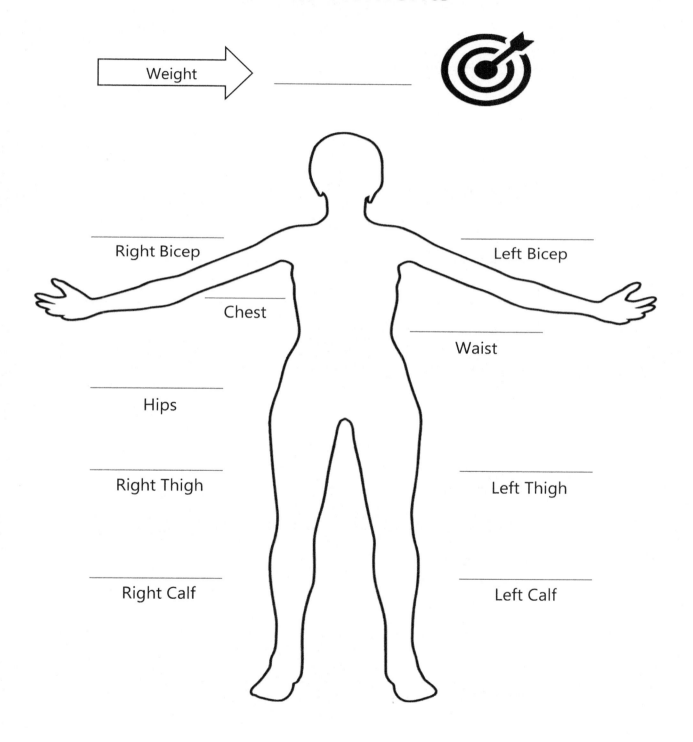

Weight _____

Right Bicep

Left Bicep

Chest

Waist

Hips

Right Thigh

Left Thigh

Right Calf

Left Calf

# Questions To Ask Yourself

Am I happy with my results after the last 7 days?

_____

_____

_____

_____

What was my biggest win?

_____

_____

_____

_____

What adjustments should I make?

_____

_____

_____

_____

How does my body feel?

_____

_____

_____

_____

# DAY 29 - 35

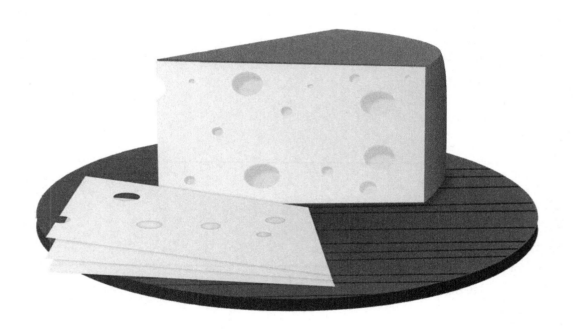

# Meal Planner

| | |
|---|---|
| Day 1 | Breakfast:<br>Lunch:<br>Dinner: |
| Day 2 | Breakfast:<br>Lunch:<br>Dinner: |
| Day 3 | Breakfast:<br>Lunch:<br>Dinner: |
| Day 4 | Breakfast:<br>Lunch:<br>Dinner: |
| Day 5 | Breakfast:<br>Lunch:<br>Dinner: |
| Day 6 | Breakfast:<br>Lunch:<br>Dinner: |
| Day 7 | Breakfast:<br>Lunch:<br>Dinner: |
| Snacks | |

# Exercise Tracker

Day 29 - 35

| Day 1 |
|---|
| |
| Cardio ◯ |
| Weights ◯ |

| Day 2 |
|---|
| |
| Cardio ◯ |
| Weights ◯ |

| Day 3 |
|---|
| |
| Cardio ◯ |
| Weights ◯ |

| Day 4 |
|---|
| |
| Cardio ◯ |
| Weights ◯ |

| Day 5 |
|---|
| |
| Cardio ◯ |
| Weights ◯ |

| Day 6 |
|---|
| |
| Cardio ◯ |
| Weights ◯ |

| Day 7 |
|---|
| |
| Cardio ◯ |
| Weights ◯ |

| Day | Calories Burned |
|---|---|
| 1 | |
| 2 | |
| 3 | |
| 4 | |
| 5 | |
| 6 | |
| 7 | |

# Day 29    Food Tracker    Date: _____
MON TUE WED THU FRI SAT SUN

| ⊕ Daily Target | | | | | | |
|---|---|---|---|---|---|---|
| **Breakfast** | Calories | Fat | Protein | Carbs | Fiber | Net Carbs |
| | | | | | | |
| | | | | | | |
| | | | | | | |
| Total: | | | | | | |
| **Lunch** | Calories | Fat | Protein | Carbs | Fiber | Net Carbs |
| | | | | | | |
| | | | | | | |
| | | | | | | |
| Total: | | | | | | |
| **Dinner** | Calories | Fat | Protein | Carbs | Fiber | Net Carbs |
| | | | | | | |
| | | | | | | |
| | | | | | | |
| Total: | | | | | | |
| **Snacks** | Calories | Fat | Protein | Carbs | Fiber | Net Carbs |
| | | | | | | |
| | | | | | | |
| | | | | | | |
| Total: | | | | | | |
| **Daily Total** | | | | | | |

**Ketosis:**   Y/N    Intermittent Fasting: From _____am/pm - To_____am/pm

# Day 30    Food Tracker

Date: _____

MON TUE WED THU FRI SAT SUN

| 🎯 Daily Target | | | | | | |
|---|---|---|---|---|---|---|
| **Breakfast** | Calories | Fat | Protein | Carbs | Fiber | Net Carbs |
| | | | | | | |
| | | | | | | |
| | | | | | | |
| | | | | | | |
| Total: | | | | | | |
| **Lunch** | Calories | Fat | Protein | Carbs | Fiber | Net Carbs |
| | | | | | | |
| | | | | | | |
| | | | | | | |
| | | | | | | |
| Total: | | | | | | |
| **Dinner** | Calories | Fat | Protein | Carbs | Fiber | Net Carbs |
| | | | | | | |
| | | | | | | |
| | | | | | | |
| | | | | | | |
| Total: | | | | | | |
| **Snacks** | Calories | Fat | Protein | Carbs | Fiber | Net Carbs |
| | | | | | | |
| | | | | | | |
| | | | | | | |
| Total: | | | | | | |
| **Daily Total** | | | | | | |

**Ketosis:**   Y/N    Intermittent Fasting: From _____am/pm - To_____am/pm

# Day 31    Food Tracker

Date: _____

MON TUE WED THU FRI SAT SUN

| 🎯 Daily Target | | | | | | |
|---|---|---|---|---|---|---|
| **Breakfast** | Calories | Fat | Protein | Carbs | Fiber | Net Carbs |
| | | | | | | |
| | | | | | | |
| | | | | | | |
| | | | | | | |
| Total: | | | | | | |
| **Lunch** | Calories | Fat | Protein | Carbs | Fiber | Net Carbs |
| | | | | | | |
| | | | | | | |
| | | | | | | |
| | | | | | | |
| Total: | | | | | | |
| **Dinner** | Calories | Fat | Protein | Carbs | Fiber | Net Carbs |
| | | | | | | |
| | | | | | | |
| | | | | | | |
| | | | | | | |
| Total: | | | | | | |
| **Snacks** | Calories | Fat | Protein | Carbs | Fiber | Net Carbs |
| | | | | | | |
| | | | | | | |
| | | | | | | |
| Total: | | | | | | |
| **Daily Total** | | | | | | |

**Ketosis:**   Y/N    Intermittent Fasting: From _____am/pm  -  To_____am/pm

# Day 32　　Food Tracker

Date: _____

| ⊕ Daily Target | | | | | | |
|---|---|---|---|---|---|---|
| **Breakfast** | Calories | Fat | Protein | Carbs | Fiber | Net Carbs |
| | | | | | | |
| | | | | | | |
| | | | | | | |
| | | | | | | |
| Total: | | | | | | |
| **Lunch** | Calories | Fat | Protein | Carbs | Fiber | Net Carbs |
| | | | | | | |
| | | | | | | |
| | | | | | | |
| | | | | | | |
| Total: | | | | | | |
| **Dinner** | Calories | Fat | Protein | Carbs | Fiber | Net Carbs |
| | | | | | | |
| | | | | | | |
| | | | | | | |
| | | | | | | |
| Total: | | | | | | |
| **Snacks** | Calories | Fat | Protein | Carbs | Fiber | Net Carbs |
| | | | | | | |
| | | | | | | |
| | | | | | | |
| Total: | | | | | | |
| **Daily Total** | | | | | | |

**Ketosis:**　Y/N　　Intermittent Fasting: From _____am/pm - To_____am/pm

# Day 33    Food Tracker

| 🎯 Daily Target | | | | | | |
|---|---|---|---|---|---|---|
| **Breakfast** | Calories | Fat | Protein | Carbs | Fiber | Net Carbs |
| | | | | | | |
| | | | | | | |
| | | | | | | |
| | | | | | | |
| Total: | | | | | | |
| **Lunch** | Calories | Fat | Protein | Carbs | Fiber | Net Carbs |
| | | | | | | |
| | | | | | | |
| | | | | | | |
| | | | | | | |
| Total: | | | | | | |
| **Dinner** | Calories | Fat | Protein | Carbs | Fiber | Net Carbs |
| | | | | | | |
| | | | | | | |
| | | | | | | |
| | | | | | | |
| Total: | | | | | | |
| **Snacks** | Calories | Fat | Protein | Carbs | Fiber | Net Carbs |
| | | | | | | |
| | | | | | | |
| | | | | | | |
| Total: | | | | | | |
| **Daily Total** | | | | | | |

**Ketosis:**   Y/N     Intermittent Fasting: From _____am/pm - To_____am/pm

# Day 34　Food Tracker

Date: _____

| ⊕ Daily Target | | | | | | |
|---|---|---|---|---|---|---|
| **Breakfast** | Calories | Fat | Protein | Carbs | Fiber | Net Carbs |
| | | | | | | |
| | | | | | | |
| | | | | | | |
| | | | | | | |
| Total: | | | | | | |
| **Lunch** | Calories | Fat | Protein | Carbs | Fiber | Net Carbs |
| | | | | | | |
| | | | | | | |
| | | | | | | |
| | | | | | | |
| Total: | | | | | | |
| **Dinner** | Calories | Fat | Protein | Carbs | Fiber | Net Carbs |
| | | | | | | |
| | | | | | | |
| | | | | | | |
| | | | | | | |
| Total: | | | | | | |
| **Snacks** | Calories | Fat | Protein | Carbs | Fiber | Net Carbs |
| | | | | | | |
| | | | | | | |
| | | | | | | |
| Total: | | | | | | |
| **Daily Total** | | | | | | |

**Ketosis:** Y/N　Intermittent Fasting: From _____am/pm - To_____am/pm

# Day 35      Food Tracker      Date: _____
MON TUE WED THU FRI SAT SUN

| ⊕ Daily Target | | | | | | |
|---|---|---|---|---|---|---|
| **Breakfast** | Calories | Fat | Protein | Carbs | Fiber | Net Carbs |
| | | | | | | |
| | | | | | | |
| | | | | | | |
| | | | | | | |
| Total: | | | | | | |
| **Lunch** | Calories | Fat | Protein | Carbs | Fiber | Net Carbs |
| | | | | | | |
| | | | | | | |
| | | | | | | |
| | | | | | | |
| | | | | | | |
| Total: | | | | | | |
| **Dinner** | Calories | Fat | Protein | Carbs | Fiber | Net Carbs |
| | | | | | | |
| | | | | | | |
| | | | | | | |
| | | | | | | |
| Total: | | | | | | |
| **Snacks** | Calories | Fat | Protein | Carbs | Fiber | Net Carbs |
| | | | | | | |
| | | | | | | |
| | | | | | | |
| Total: | | | | | | |
| **Daily Total** | | | | | | |

**Ketosis:**   Y/N      Intermittent Fasting: From _____am/pm  -  To_____am/pm

# NOTES

# DAY 36 – WEIGHT

## Measurements

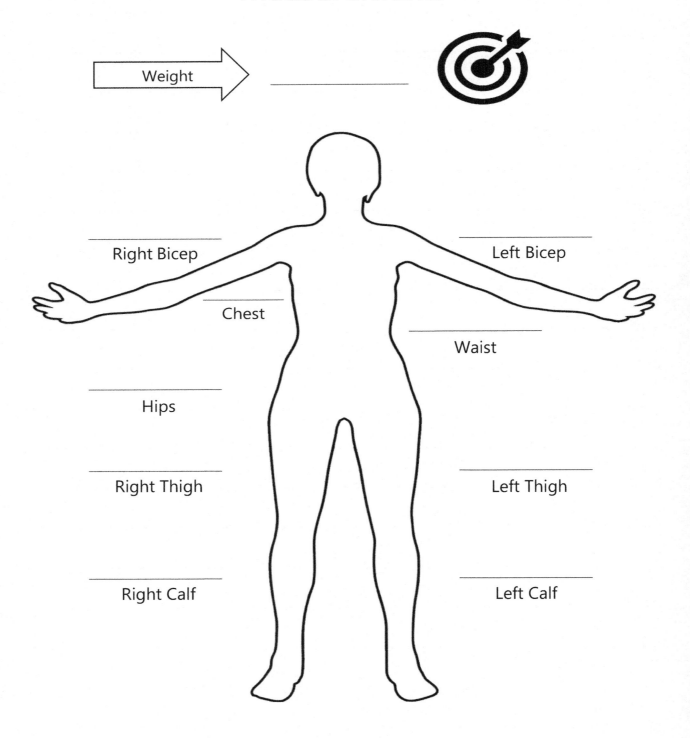

Weight ⟶ _____

Right Bicep _____

Left Bicep _____

Chest _____

Waist _____

Hips _____

Right Thigh _____

Left Thigh _____

Right Calf _____

Left Calf _____

# Questions To Ask Yourself

Am I happy with my results after the last 7 days?

_____

_____

_____

_____

What was my biggest win?

_____

_____

_____

_____

What adjustments should I make?

_____

_____

_____

_____

How does my body feel?

_____

_____

_____

_____

# DAY 36 - 42

# Meal Planner

| | |
|---|---|
| Day 1 | Breakfast:<br><br>Lunch:<br><br>Dinner: |
| Day 2 | Breakfast:<br><br>Lunch:<br><br>Dinner: |
| Day 3 | Breakfast:<br><br>Lunch:<br><br>Dinner: |
| Day 4 | Breakfast:<br><br>Lunch:<br><br>Dinner: |
| Day 5 | Breakfast:<br><br>Lunch:<br><br>Dinner: |
| Day 6 | Breakfast:<br><br>Lunch:<br><br>Dinner: |
| Day 7 | Breakfast:<br><br>Lunch:<br><br>Dinner: |
| Snacks | |

# Exercise Tracker

| Day 1 |
|---|
| |

Cardio ○
Weights ○

| Day 2 |
|---|
| |

Cardio ○
Weights ○

| Day 3 |
|---|
| |

Cardio ○
Weights ○

| Day 4 |
|---|
| |

Cardio ○
Weights ○

| Day 5 |
|---|
| |

Cardio ○
Weights ○

| Day 6 |
|---|
| |

Cardio ○
Weights ○

| Day 7 |
|---|
| |

Cardio ○
Weights ○

| Day | Calories Burned |
|---|---|
| 1 | |
| 2 | |
| 3 | |
| 4 | |
| 5 | |
| 6 | |
| 7 | |

# Day 36     Food Tracker     Date: _____

MON TUE WED THU FRI SAT SUN

| 🎯 **Daily Target** | | | | | | |
|---|---|---|---|---|---|---|
| **Breakfast** | Calories | Fat | Protein | Carbs | Fiber | Net Carbs |
| | | | | | | |
| | | | | | | |
| | | | | | | |
| | | | | | | |
| Total: | | | | | | |
| **Lunch** | Calories | Fat | Protein | Carbs | Fiber | Net Carbs |
| | | | | | | |
| | | | | | | |
| | | | | | | |
| | | | | | | |
| Total: | | | | | | |
| **Dinner** | Calories | Fat | Protein | Carbs | Fiber | Net Carbs |
| | | | | | | |
| | | | | | | |
| | | | | | | |
| | | | | | | |
| Total: | | | | | | |
| **Snacks** | Calories | Fat | Protein | Carbs | Fiber | Net Carbs |
| | | | | | | |
| | | | | | | |
| | | | | | | |
| Total: | | | | | | |
| **Daily Total** | | | | | | |

**Ketosis:**   Y/N     Intermittent Fasting: From _____am/pm - To_____am/pm

# Day 37    Food Tracker    Date: _____
MON TUE WED THU FRI SAT SUN

| 🎯 Daily Target | | | | | | |
|---|---|---|---|---|---|---|
| **Breakfast** | Calories | Fat | Protein | Carbs | Fiber | Net Carbs |
| | | | | | | |
| | | | | | | |
| | | | | | | |
| | | | | | | |
| Total: | | | | | | |
| **Lunch** | Calories | Fat | Protein | Carbs | Fiber | Net Carbs |
| | | | | | | |
| | | | | | | |
| | | | | | | |
| | | | | | | |
| Total: | | | | | | |
| **Dinner** | Calories | Fat | Protein | Carbs | Fiber | Net Carbs |
| | | | | | | |
| | | | | | | |
| | | | | | | |
| | | | | | | |
| Total: | | | | | | |
| **Snacks** | Calories | Fat | Protein | Carbs | Fiber | Net Carbs |
| | | | | | | |
| | | | | | | |
| | | | | | | |
| Total: | | | | | | |
| **Daily Total** | | | | | | |

**Ketosis:**   Y/N    Intermittent Fasting: From _____am/pm - To_____am/pm

# Day 38    Food Tracker

Date: _____

MON TUE WED THU FRI SAT SUN

| ⊕ Daily Target | | | | | | |
|---|---|---|---|---|---|---|
| **Breakfast** | Calories | Fat | Protein | Carbs | Fiber | Net Carbs |
| | | | | | | |
| | | | | | | |
| | | | | | | |
| Total: | | | | | | |
| **Lunch** | Calories | Fat | Protein | Carbs | Fiber | Net Carbs |
| | | | | | | |
| | | | | | | |
| | | | | | | |
| Total: | | | | | | |
| **Dinner** | Calories | Fat | Protein | Carbs | Fiber | Net Carbs |
| | | | | | | |
| | | | | | | |
| | | | | | | |
| Total: | | | | | | |
| **Snacks** | Calories | Fat | Protein | Carbs | Fiber | Net Carbs |
| | | | | | | |
| | | | | | | |
| Total: | | | | | | |
| **Daily Total** | | | | | | |

**Ketosis:**   Y/N    Intermittent Fasting: From _____am/pm - To_____am/pm

# Day 39    Food Tracker

Date: _____
MON TUE WED THU FRI SAT SUN

| 🎯 Daily Target | | | | | | |
|---|---|---|---|---|---|---|
| **Breakfast** | Calories | Fat | Protein | Carbs | Fiber | Net Carbs |
| | | | | | | |
| | | | | | | |
| | | | | | | |
| | | | | | | |
| Total: | | | | | | |
| **Lunch** | Calories | Fat | Protein | Carbs | Fiber | Net Carbs |
| | | | | | | |
| | | | | | | |
| | | | | | | |
| | | | | | | |
| Total: | | | | | | |
| **Dinner** | Calories | Fat | Protein | Carbs | Fiber | Net Carbs |
| | | | | | | |
| | | | | | | |
| | | | | | | |
| | | | | | | |
| Total: | | | | | | |
| **Snacks** | Calories | Fat | Protein | Carbs | Fiber | Net Carbs |
| | | | | | | |
| | | | | | | |
| | | | | | | |
| Total: | | | | | | |
| **Daily Total** | | | | | | |

**Ketosis:**  Y/N     **Intermittent Fasting: From** _____am/pm - **To**_____am/pm

# Day 40  Food Tracker

Date: _____

| ⊕ Daily Target | | | | | | |
|---|---|---|---|---|---|---|
| **Breakfast** | Calories | Fat | Protein | Carbs | Fiber | Net Carbs |
| | | | | | | |
| | | | | | | |
| | | | | | | |
| | | | | | | |
| Total: | | | | | | |
| **Lunch** | Calories | Fat | Protein | Carbs | Fiber | Net Carbs |
| | | | | | | |
| | | | | | | |
| | | | | | | |
| | | | | | | |
| Total: | | | | | | |
| **Dinner** | Calories | Fat | Protein | Carbs | Fiber | Net Carbs |
| | | | | | | |
| | | | | | | |
| | | | | | | |
| | | | | | | |
| Total: | | | | | | |
| **Snacks** | Calories | Fat | Protein | Carbs | Fiber | Net Carbs |
| | | | | | | |
| | | | | | | |
| | | | | | | |
| Total: | | | | | | |
| **Daily Total** | | | | | | |

**Ketosis:**   Y/N      Intermittent Fasting: From _____am/pm - To_____am/pm

# Day 41    Food Tracker

| 🎯 **Daily Target** | | | | | | |
|---|---|---|---|---|---|---|
| **Breakfast** | Calories | Fat | Protein | Carbs | Fiber | Net Carbs |
| | | | | | | |
| | | | | | | |
| | | | | | | |
| | | | | | | |
| Total: | | | | | | |
| **Lunch** | Calories | Fat | Protein | Carbs | Fiber | Net Carbs |
| | | | | | | |
| | | | | | | |
| | | | | | | |
| | | | | | | |
| Total: | | | | | | |
| **Dinner** | Calories | Fat | Protein | Carbs | Fiber | Net Carbs |
| | | | | | | |
| | | | | | | |
| | | | | | | |
| | | | | | | |
| Total: | | | | | | |
| **Snacks** | Calories | Fat | Protein | Carbs | Fiber | Net Carbs |
| | | | | | | |
| | | | | | | |
| | | | | | | |
| Total: | | | | | | |
| **Daily Total** | | | | | | |

**Ketosis:**   Y/N     Intermittent Fasting: From _____am/pm  -  To_____am/pm

# Day 42      Food Tracker      Date: _____

| ⊕ Daily Target | | | | | | |
|---|---|---|---|---|---|---|
| **Breakfast** | Calories | Fat | Protein | Carbs | Fiber | Net Carbs |
| | | | | | | |
| | | | | | | |
| | | | | | | |
| | | | | | | |
| Total: | | | | | | |
| **Lunch** | Calories | Fat | Protein | Carbs | Fiber | Net Carbs |
| | | | | | | |
| | | | | | | |
| | | | | | | |
| | | | | | | |
| Total: | | | | | | |
| **Dinner** | Calories | Fat | Protein | Carbs | Fiber | Net Carbs |
| | | | | | | |
| | | | | | | |
| | | | | | | |
| | | | | | | |
| Total: | | | | | | |
| **Snacks** | Calories | Fat | Protein | Carbs | Fiber | Net Carbs |
| | | | | | | |
| | | | | | | |
| | | | | | | |
| Total: | | | | | | |
| **Daily Total** | | | | | | |

**Ketosis:**   Y/N      Intermittent Fasting: From _____am/pm  -  To_____am/pm

# NOTES

# DAY 43 – WEIGHT

## Measurements

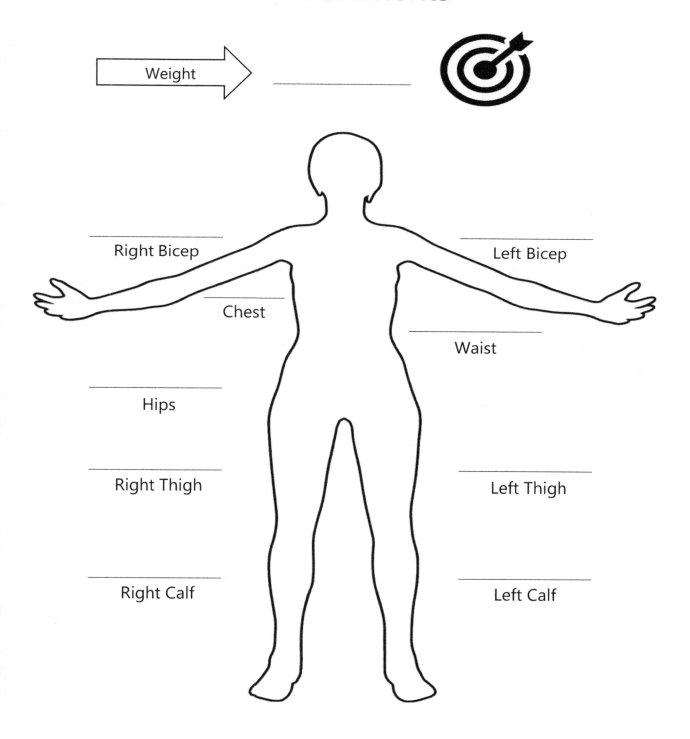

Weight ⟶ _____

Right Bicep _____

Left Bicep _____

Chest _____

Waist _____

Hips _____

Right Thigh _____

Left Thigh _____

Right Calf _____

Left Calf _____

# Questions To Ask Yourself

Am I happy with my results after the last 7 days?

_____

_____

_____

_____

What was my biggest win?

_____

_____

_____

_____

What adjustments should I make?

_____

_____

_____

_____

How does my body feel?

_____

_____

_____

_____

# DAY 43 - 49

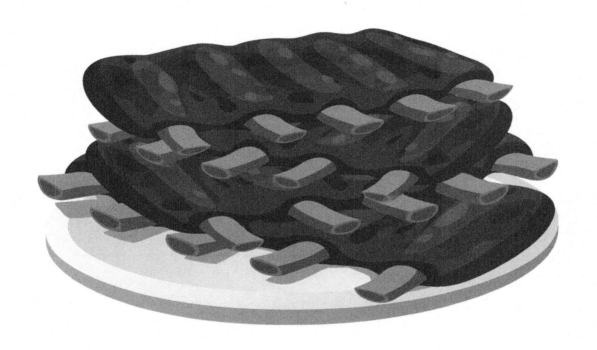

# Meal Planner

| | |
|---|---|
| **Day 1** | Breakfast:<br>Lunch:<br>Dinner: |
| **Day 2** | Breakfast:<br>Lunch:<br>Dinner: |
| **Day 3** | Breakfast:<br>Lunch:<br>Dinner: |
| **Day 4** | Breakfast:<br>Lunch:<br>Dinner: |
| **Day 5** | Breakfast:<br>Lunch:<br>Dinner: |
| **Day 6** | Breakfast:<br>Lunch:<br>Dinner: |
| **Day 7** | Breakfast:<br>Lunch:<br>Dinner: |
| **Snacks** | |

# Exercise Tracker

Day 43 - 49

| Day 1 |
|---|
| |
| Cardio ◯ |
| Weights ◯ |

| Day 2 |
|---|
| |
| Cardio ◯ |
| Weights ◯ |

| Day 3 |
|---|
| |
| Cardio ◯ |
| Weights ◯ |

| Day 4 |
|---|
| |
| Cardio ◯ |
| Weights ◯ |

| Day 5 |
|---|
| |
| Cardio ◯ |
| Weights ◯ |

| Day 6 |
|---|
| |
| Cardio ◯ |
| Weights ◯ |

| Day 7 |
|---|
| |
| Cardio ◯ |
| Weights ◯ |

| Day | Calories Burned |
|---|---|
| 1 | |
| 2 | |
| 3 | |
| 4 | |
| 5 | |
| 6 | |
| 7 | |

# Day 43    Food Tracker

| 🎯 Daily Target | | | | | | |
|---|---|---|---|---|---|---|
| **Breakfast** | Calories | Fat | Protein | Carbs | Fiber | Net Carbs |
| | | | | | | |
| | | | | | | |
| | | | | | | |
| | | | | | | |
| Total: | | | | | | |
| **Lunch** | Calories | Fat | Protein | Carbs | Fiber | Net Carbs |
| | | | | | | |
| | | | | | | |
| | | | | | | |
| | | | | | | |
| Total: | | | | | | |
| **Dinner** | Calories | Fat | Protein | Carbs | Fiber | Net Carbs |
| | | | | | | |
| | | | | | | |
| | | | | | | |
| | | | | | | |
| Total: | | | | | | |
| **Snacks** | Calories | Fat | Protein | Carbs | Fiber | Net Carbs |
| | | | | | | |
| | | | | | | |
| | | | | | | |
| Total: | | | | | | |
| **Daily Total** | | | | | | |

**Ketosis:**   Y/N    Intermittent Fasting: From _____am/pm - To_____am/pm

# Day 44    Food Tracker    Date: _____

| 🎯 Daily Target | | | | | | |
|---|---|---|---|---|---|---|
| **Breakfast** | Calories | Fat | Protein | Carbs | Fiber | Net Carbs |
| | | | | | | |
| | | | | | | |
| | | | | | | |
| | | | | | | |
| Total: | | | | | | |
| **Lunch** | Calories | Fat | Protein | Carbs | Fiber | Net Carbs |
| | | | | | | |
| | | | | | | |
| | | | | | | |
| | | | | | | |
| Total: | | | | | | |
| **Dinner** | Calories | Fat | Protein | Carbs | Fiber | Net Carbs |
| | | | | | | |
| | | | | | | |
| | | | | | | |
| | | | | | | |
| Total: | | | | | | |
| **Snacks** | Calories | Fat | Protein | Carbs | Fiber | Net Carbs |
| | | | | | | |
| | | | | | | |
| | | | | | | |
| Total: | | | | | | |
| **Daily Total** | | | | | | |

**Ketosis:**   Y/N    Intermittent Fasting: From _____am/pm - To_____am/pm

# Day 45    Food Tracker

Date: _____

MON TUE WED THU FRI SAT SUN

| 🎯 Daily Target | | | | | | |
|---|---|---|---|---|---|---|

| **Breakfast** | Calories | Fat | Protein | Carbs | Fiber | Net Carbs |
|---|---|---|---|---|---|---|
| | | | | | | |
| | | | | | | |
| | | | | | | |
| | | | | | | |
| Total: | | | | | | |

| **Lunch** | Calories | Fat | Protein | Carbs | Fiber | Net Carbs |
|---|---|---|---|---|---|---|
| | | | | | | |
| | | | | | | |
| | | | | | | |
| | | | | | | |
| Total: | | | | | | |

| **Dinner** | Calories | Fat | Protein | Carbs | Fiber | Net Carbs |
|---|---|---|---|---|---|---|
| | | | | | | |
| | | | | | | |
| | | | | | | |
| | | | | | | |
| Total: | | | | | | |

| **Snacks** | Calories | Fat | Protein | Carbs | Fiber | Net Carbs |
|---|---|---|---|---|---|---|
| | | | | | | |
| | | | | | | |
| | | | | | | |
| Total: | | | | | | |

| **Daily Total** | | | | | | |
|---|---|---|---|---|---|---|

**Ketosis:** Y/N    Intermittent Fasting: From _____am/pm - To_____am/pm

# Day 46    Food Tracker

| 🎯 **Daily Target** | | | | | | |
|---|---|---|---|---|---|---|
| **Breakfast** | Calories | Fat | Protein | Carbs | Fiber | Net Carbs |
| | | | | | | |
| | | | | | | |
| | | | | | | |
| | | | | | | |
| Total: | | | | | | |
| **Lunch** | Calories | Fat | Protein | Carbs | Fiber | Net Carbs |
| | | | | | | |
| | | | | | | |
| | | | | | | |
| | | | | | | |
| Total: | | | | | | |
| **Dinner** | Calories | Fat | Protein | Carbs | Fiber | Net Carbs |
| | | | | | | |
| | | | | | | |
| | | | | | | |
| | | | | | | |
| Total: | | | | | | |
| **Snacks** | Calories | Fat | Protein | Carbs | Fiber | Net Carbs |
| | | | | | | |
| | | | | | | |
| | | | | | | |
| Total: | | | | | | |
| **Daily Total** | | | | | | |

**Ketosis:**   Y/N    Intermittent Fasting: From _____am/pm - To_____am/pm

# Day 47    Food Tracker    Date: _____
MON TUE WED THU FRI SAT SUN

| 🎯 Daily Target | | | | | | |
|---|---|---|---|---|---|---|
| **Breakfast** | Calories | Fat | Protein | Carbs | Fiber | Net Carbs |
| | | | | | | |
| | | | | | | |
| | | | | | | |
| | | | | | | |
| Total: | | | | | | |
| **Lunch** | Calories | Fat | Protein | Carbs | Fiber | Net Carbs |
| | | | | | | |
| | | | | | | |
| | | | | | | |
| | | | | | | |
| Total: | | | | | | |
| **Dinner** | Calories | Fat | Protein | Carbs | Fiber | Net Carbs |
| | | | | | | |
| | | | | | | |
| | | | | | | |
| | | | | | | |
| Total: | | | | | | |
| **Snacks** | Calories | Fat | Protein | Carbs | Fiber | Net Carbs |
| | | | | | | |
| | | | | | | |
| | | | | | | |
| Total: | | | | | | |
| **Daily Total** | | | | | | |

**Ketosis:**   Y/N     Intermittent Fasting: From _____am/pm  -  To_____am/pm

# Day 48    Food Tracker    Date: _____

| ⊕ Daily Target | | | | | | |
|---|---|---|---|---|---|---|
| **Breakfast** | Calories | Fat | Protein | Carbs | Fiber | Net Carbs |
| | | | | | | |
| | | | | | | |
| | | | | | | |
| Total: | | | | | | |
| **Lunch** | Calories | Fat | Protein | Carbs | Fiber | Net Carbs |
| | | | | | | |
| | | | | | | |
| | | | | | | |
| Total: | | | | | | |
| **Dinner** | Calories | Fat | Protein | Carbs | Fiber | Net Carbs |
| | | | | | | |
| | | | | | | |
| | | | | | | |
| Total: | | | | | | |
| **Snacks** | Calories | Fat | Protein | Carbs | Fiber | Net Carbs |
| | | | | | | |
| | | | | | | |
| Total: | | | | | | |
| **Daily Total** | | | | | | |

**Ketosis:**   Y/N    Intermittent Fasting: From _____am/pm - To_____am/pm

# Day 49    Food Tracker    Date: _____

| 🎯 Daily Target | | | | | | |
|---|---|---|---|---|---|---|
| **Breakfast** | Calories | Fat | Protein | Carbs | Fiber | Net Carbs |
| | | | | | | |
| | | | | | | |
| | | | | | | |
| | | | | | | |
| Total: | | | | | | |
| **Lunch** | Calories | Fat | Protein | Carbs | Fiber | Net Carbs |
| | | | | | | |
| | | | | | | |
| | | | | | | |
| | | | | | | |
| Total: | | | | | | |
| **Dinner** | Calories | Fat | Protein | Carbs | Fiber | Net Carbs |
| | | | | | | |
| | | | | | | |
| | | | | | | |
| | | | | | | |
| Total: | | | | | | |
| **Snacks** | Calories | Fat | Protein | Carbs | Fiber | Net Carbs |
| | | | | | | |
| | | | | | | |
| | | | | | | |
| Total: | | | | | | |
| **Daily Total** | | | | | | |

**Ketosis:**   Y/N      Intermittent Fasting: From _____am/pm  -  To_____am/pm

# NOTES

# DAY 50 – WEIGHT

## Measurements

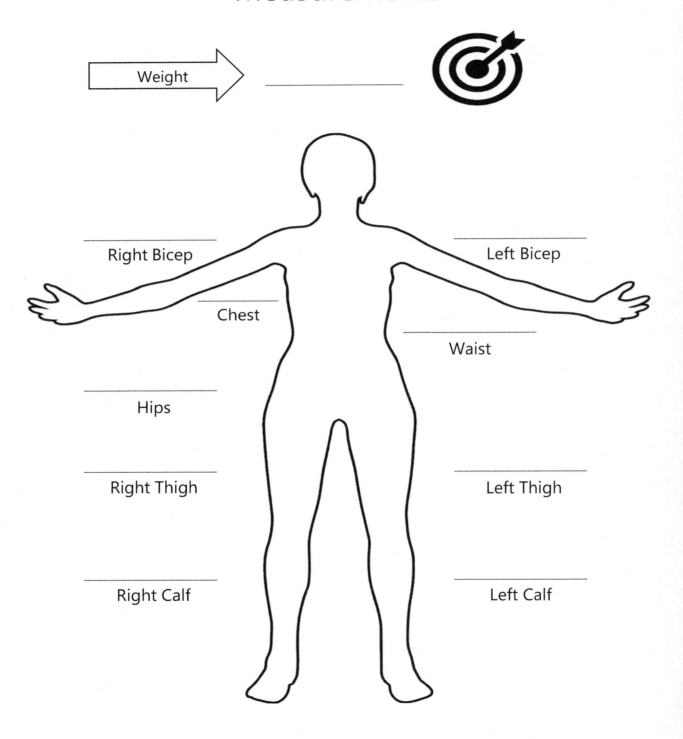

Weight ⟶ _____

Right Bicep _____

Left Bicep _____

Chest _____

Waist _____

Hips _____

Right Thigh _____

Left Thigh _____

Right Calf _____

Left Calf _____

# Questions To Ask Yourself

Am I happy with my results after the last 7 days?

_____

_____

_____

_____

What was my biggest win?

_____

_____

_____

_____

What adjustments should I make?

_____

_____

_____

_____

How does my body feel?

_____

_____

_____

_____

# DAY 50 - 56

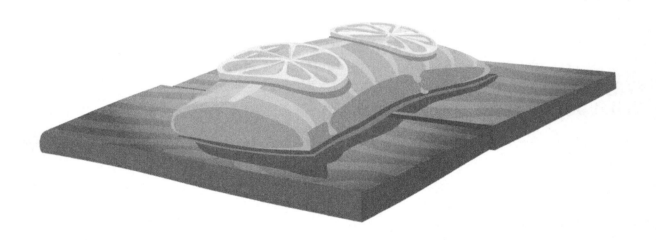

# Meal Planner

Day 50 - 56

| | |
|---|---|
| **Day 1** | Breakfast:<br>Lunch:<br>Dinner: |
| **Day 2** | Breakfast:<br>Lunch:<br>Dinner: |
| **Day 3** | Breakfast:<br>Lunch:<br>Dinner: |
| **Day 4** | Breakfast:<br>Lunch:<br>Dinner: |
| **Day 5** | Breakfast:<br>Lunch:<br>Dinner: |
| **Day 6** | Breakfast:<br>Lunch:<br>Dinner: |
| **Day 7** | Breakfast:<br>Lunch:<br>Dinner: |
| **Snacks** | |

# Exercise Tracker

| Day 1 | Day 2 | Day 3 |
|---|---|---|
| | | |

| | | |
|---|---|---|
| Cardio ○ | Cardio ○ | Cardio ○ |
| Weights ○ | Weights ○ | Weights ○ |

| Day 4 | Day 5 | Day 6 |
|---|---|---|
| | | |

| | | |
|---|---|---|
| Cardio ○ | Cardio ○ | Cardio ○ |
| Weights ○ | Weights ○ | Weights ○ |

| Day 7 |
|---|
| |

| Cardio ○ |
| Weights ○ |

| Day | Calories Burned |
|---|---|
| 1 | |
| 2 | |
| 3 | |
| 4 | |
| 5 | |
| 6 | |
| 7 | |

# Day 50    Food Tracker

| 🎯 Daily Target | | | | | | |
|---|---|---|---|---|---|---|
| **Breakfast** | Calories | Fat | Protein | Carbs | Fiber | Net Carbs |
| | | | | | | |
| | | | | | | |
| | | | | | | |
| Total: | | | | | | |
| **Lunch** | Calories | Fat | Protein | Carbs | Fiber | Net Carbs |
| | | | | | | |
| | | | | | | |
| | | | | | | |
| | | | | | | |
| Total: | | | | | | |
| **Dinner** | Calories | Fat | Protein | Carbs | Fiber | Net Carbs |
| | | | | | | |
| | | | | | | |
| | | | | | | |
| | | | | | | |
| Total: | | | | | | |
| **Snacks** | Calories | Fat | Protein | Carbs | Fiber | Net Carbs |
| | | | | | | |
| | | | | | | |
| | | | | | | |
| Total: | | | | | | |
| **Daily Total** | | | | | | |

**Ketosis:**   Y/N    Intermittent Fasting: From _____am/pm - To_____am/pm

# Day 51    Food Tracker

Date: _____

| 🎯 Daily Target | | | | | | |
|---|---|---|---|---|---|---|
| **Breakfast** | Calories | Fat | Protein | Carbs | Fiber | Net Carbs |
| | | | | | | |
| | | | | | | |
| | | | | | | |
| | | | | | | |
| Total: | | | | | | |
| **Lunch** | Calories | Fat | Protein | Carbs | Fiber | Net Carbs |
| | | | | | | |
| | | | | | | |
| | | | | | | |
| | | | | | | |
| Total: | | | | | | |
| **Dinner** | Calories | Fat | Protein | Carbs | Fiber | Net Carbs |
| | | | | | | |
| | | | | | | |
| | | | | | | |
| | | | | | | |
| Total: | | | | | | |
| **Snacks** | Calories | Fat | Protein | Carbs | Fiber | Net Carbs |
| | | | | | | |
| | | | | | | |
| | | | | | | |
| Total: | | | | | | |
| **Daily Total** | | | | | | |

**Ketosis:**   Y/N     Intermittent Fasting: From _____am/pm - To_____am/pm

# Day 52     Food Tracker     Date: _____

| ⊕ Daily Target | | | | | | |
|---|---|---|---|---|---|---|
| **Breakfast** | Calories | Fat | Protein | Carbs | Fiber | Net Carbs |
| | | | | | | |
| | | | | | | |
| | | | | | | |
| | | | | | | |
| Total: | | | | | | |
| **Lunch** | Calories | Fat | Protein | Carbs | Fiber | Net Carbs |
| | | | | | | |
| | | | | | | |
| | | | | | | |
| | | | | | | |
| Total: | | | | | | |
| **Dinner** | Calories | Fat | Protein | Carbs | Fiber | Net Carbs |
| | | | | | | |
| | | | | | | |
| | | | | | | |
| | | | | | | |
| Total: | | | | | | |
| **Snacks** | Calories | Fat | Protein | Carbs | Fiber | Net Carbs |
| | | | | | | |
| | | | | | | |
| | | | | | | |
| Total: | | | | | | |
| **Daily Total** | | | | | | |

**Ketosis:**   Y/N     Intermittent Fasting: From _____am/pm - To_____am/pm

# Day 53    Food Tracker    Date: _____

| ⊕ Daily Target | | | | | | |
|---|---|---|---|---|---|---|
| **Breakfast** | Calories | Fat | Protein | Carbs | Fiber | Net Carbs |
| | | | | | | |
| | | | | | | |
| | | | | | | |
| | | | | | | |
| Total: | | | | | | |
| **Lunch** | Calories | Fat | Protein | Carbs | Fiber | Net Carbs |
| | | | | | | |
| | | | | | | |
| | | | | | | |
| | | | | | | |
| Total: | | | | | | |
| **Dinner** | Calories | Fat | Protein | Carbs | Fiber | Net Carbs |
| | | | | | | |
| | | | | | | |
| | | | | | | |
| | | | | | | |
| Total: | | | | | | |
| **Snacks** | Calories | Fat | Protein | Carbs | Fiber | Net Carbs |
| | | | | | | |
| | | | | | | |
| | | | | | | |
| Total: | | | | | | |
| **Daily Total** | | | | | | |

**Ketosis:**    Y/N    Intermittent Fasting: From _____am/pm - To_____am/pm

# Day 54    Food Tracker

| 🎯 Daily Target | | | | | | |
|---|---|---|---|---|---|---|
| **Breakfast** | Calories | Fat | Protein | Carbs | Fiber | Net Carbs |
| | | | | | | |
| | | | | | | |
| | | | | | | |
| Total: | | | | | | |
| **Lunch** | Calories | Fat | Protein | Carbs | Fiber | Net Carbs |
| | | | | | | |
| | | | | | | |
| | | | | | | |
| Total: | | | | | | |
| **Dinner** | Calories | Fat | Protein | Carbs | Fiber | Net Carbs |
| | | | | | | |
| | | | | | | |
| | | | | | | |
| Total: | | | | | | |
| **Snacks** | Calories | Fat | Protein | Carbs | Fiber | Net Carbs |
| | | | | | | |
| | | | | | | |
| | | | | | | |
| Total: | | | | | | |
| **Daily Total** | | | | | | |

**Ketosis:**   Y/N    Intermittent Fasting: From _____am/pm - To_____am/pm

# Day 55    Food Tracker    Date: _____

| ⊕ Daily Target | | | | | | |
|---|---|---|---|---|---|---|
| **Breakfast** | Calories | Fat | Protein | Carbs | Fiber | Net Carbs |
| | | | | | | |
| | | | | | | |
| | | | | | | |
| | | | | | | |
| Total: | | | | | | |
| **Lunch** | Calories | Fat | Protein | Carbs | Fiber | Net Carbs |
| | | | | | | |
| | | | | | | |
| | | | | | | |
| | | | | | | |
| Total: | | | | | | |
| **Dinner** | Calories | Fat | Protein | Carbs | Fiber | Net Carbs |
| | | | | | | |
| | | | | | | |
| | | | | | | |
| | | | | | | |
| Total: | | | | | | |
| **Snacks** | Calories | Fat | Protein | Carbs | Fiber | Net Carbs |
| | | | | | | |
| | | | | | | |
| | | | | | | |
| Total: | | | | | | |
| **Daily Total** | | | | | | |

**Ketosis:**    Y/N    Intermittent Fasting: From _____am/pm - To_____am/pm

# Day 56    Food Tracker    Date: _____
MON TUE WED THU FRI SAT SUN

| ⊕ Daily Target | | | | | | |
|---|---|---|---|---|---|---|
| **Breakfast** | Calories | Fat | Protein | Carbs | Fiber | Net Carbs |
| | | | | | | |
| | | | | | | |
| | | | | | | |
| | | | | | | |
| Total: | | | | | | |
| **Lunch** | Calories | Fat | Protein | Carbs | Fiber | Net Carbs |
| | | | | | | |
| | | | | | | |
| | | | | | | |
| | | | | | | |
| Total: | | | | | | |
| **Dinner** | Calories | Fat | Protein | Carbs | Fiber | Net Carbs |
| | | | | | | |
| | | | | | | |
| | | | | | | |
| | | | | | | |
| Total: | | | | | | |
| **Snacks** | Calories | Fat | Protein | Carbs | Fiber | Net Carbs |
| | | | | | | |
| | | | | | | |
| | | | | | | |
| Total: | | | | | | |
| **Daily Total** | | | | | | |

**Ketosis:**    Y/N        Intermittent Fasting: From _____am/pm  -  To_____am/pm

# NOTES

# DAY 57 – WEIGHT

## Measurements

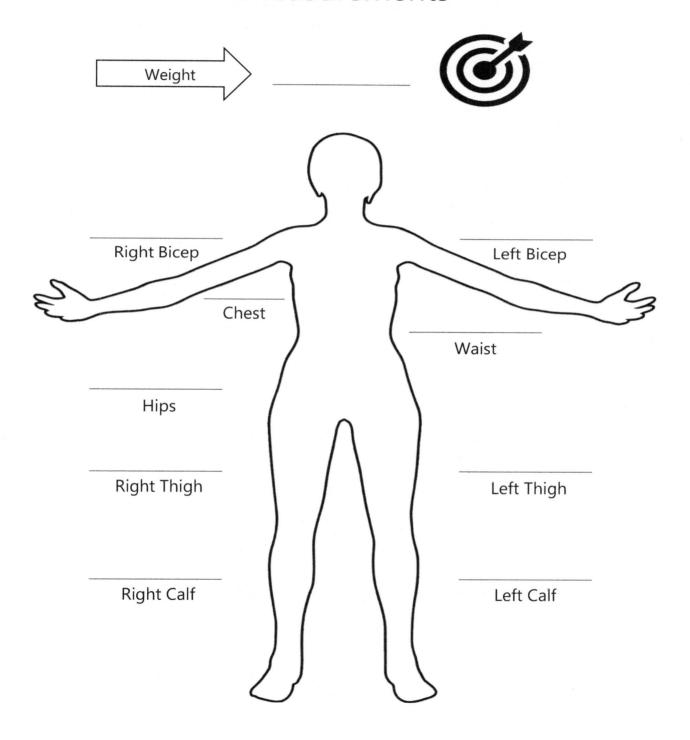

Weight _____

Right Bicep _____

Left Bicep _____

Chest _____

Waist _____

Hips _____

Right Thigh _____

Left Thigh _____

Right Calf _____

Left Calf _____

# Questions To Ask Yourself

Am I happy with my results after the last 7 days?

_____

_____

_____

_____

What was my biggest win?

_____

_____

_____

_____

What adjustments should I make?

_____

_____

_____

_____

How does my body feel?

_____

_____

_____

_____

# DAY 57 - 63

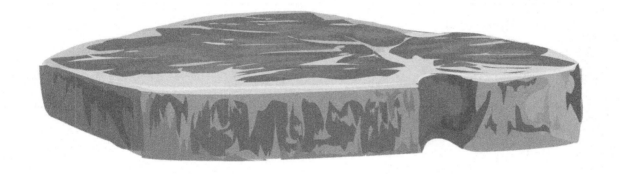

# Meal Planner

| | |
|---|---|
| Day 1 | Breakfast:<br>Lunch:<br>Dinner: |
| Day 2 | Breakfast:<br>Lunch:<br>Dinner: |
| Day 3 | Breakfast:<br>Lunch:<br>Dinner: |
| Day 4 | Breakfast:<br>Lunch:<br>Dinner: |
| Day 5 | Breakfast:<br>Lunch:<br>Dinner: |
| Day 6 | Breakfast:<br>Lunch:<br>Dinner: |
| Day 7 | Breakfast:<br>Lunch:<br>Dinner: |
| Snacks | |

# Exercise Tracker

Day 57 - 63

| Day 1 | Day 2 | Day 3 |
|---|---|---|
| | | |
| Cardio ◯ <br> Weights ◯ | Cardio ◯ <br> Weights ◯ | Cardio ◯ <br> Weights ◯ |

| Day 4 | Day 5 | Day 6 |
|---|---|---|
| | | |
| Cardio ◯ <br> Weights ◯ | Cardio ◯ <br> Weights ◯ | Cardio ◯ <br> Weights ◯ |

| Day 7 |
|---|
| |
| Cardio ◯ <br> Weights ◯ |

| Day | Calories Burned |
|---|---|
| 1 | |
| 2 | |
| 3 | |
| 4 | |
| 5 | |
| 6 | |
| 7 | |

# Day 57    Food Tracker

Date: _____
MON TUE WED THU FRI SAT SUN

| 🎯 Daily Target | | | | | | |
|---|---|---|---|---|---|---|
| **Breakfast** | Calories | Fat | Protein | Carbs | Fiber | Net Carbs |
| | | | | | | |
| | | | | | | |
| | | | | | | |
| | | | | | | |
| Total: | | | | | | |
| **Lunch** | Calories | Fat | Protein | Carbs | Fiber | Net Carbs |
| | | | | | | |
| | | | | | | |
| | | | | | | |
| | | | | | | |
| Total: | | | | | | |
| **Dinner** | Calories | Fat | Protein | Carbs | Fiber | Net Carbs |
| | | | | | | |
| | | | | | | |
| | | | | | | |
| | | | | | | |
| Total: | | | | | | |
| **Snacks** | Calories | Fat | Protein | Carbs | Fiber | Net Carbs |
| | | | | | | |
| | | | | | | |
| | | | | | | |
| Total: | | | | | | |
| **Daily Total** | | | | | | |

**Ketosis:**   Y/N     Intermittent Fasting: From _____am/pm - To_____am/pm

# Day 58    Food Tracker    Date: _____

| 🎯 Daily Target | | | | | | |
|---|---|---|---|---|---|---|
| **Breakfast** | Calories | Fat | Protein | Carbs | Fiber | Net Carbs |
| | | | | | | |
| | | | | | | |
| | | | | | | |
| Total: | | | | | | |
| **Lunch** | Calories | Fat | Protein | Carbs | Fiber | Net Carbs |
| | | | | | | |
| | | | | | | |
| | | | | | | |
| | | | | | | |
| Total: | | | | | | |
| **Dinner** | Calories | Fat | Protein | Carbs | Fiber | Net Carbs |
| | | | | | | |
| | | | | | | |
| | | | | | | |
| | | | | | | |
| Total: | | | | | | |
| **Snacks** | Calories | Fat | Protein | Carbs | Fiber | Net Carbs |
| | | | | | | |
| | | | | | | |
| | | | | | | |
| Total: | | | | | | |
| **Daily Total** | | | | | | |

**Ketosis:**   Y/N    Intermittent Fasting: From _____am/pm - To_____am/pm

# Day 59     Food Tracker

Date: _____
MON TUE WED THU FRI SAT SUN

| 🎯 Daily Target | | | | | | |
|---|---|---|---|---|---|---|
| **Breakfast** | Calories | Fat | Protein | Carbs | Fiber | Net Carbs |
| | | | | | | |
| | | | | | | |
| | | | | | | |
| | | | | | | |
| Total: | | | | | | |
| **Lunch** | Calories | Fat | Protein | Carbs | Fiber | Net Carbs |
| | | | | | | |
| | | | | | | |
| | | | | | | |
| | | | | | | |
| Total: | | | | | | |
| **Dinner** | Calories | Fat | Protein | Carbs | Fiber | Net Carbs |
| | | | | | | |
| | | | | | | |
| | | | | | | |
| | | | | | | |
| Total: | | | | | | |
| **Snacks** | Calories | Fat | Protein | Carbs | Fiber | Net Carbs |
| | | | | | | |
| | | | | | | |
| | | | | | | |
| Total: | | | | | | |
| **Daily Total** | | | | | | |

**Ketosis:**   Y/N     Intermittent Fasting: From _____am/pm - To_____am/pm

# Day 60    Food Tracker

| 🎯 Daily Target | | | | | | |
|---|---|---|---|---|---|---|
| **Breakfast** | Calories | Fat | Protein | Carbs | Fiber | Net Carbs |
| | | | | | | |
| | | | | | | |
| | | | | | | |
| Total: | | | | | | |
| **Lunch** | Calories | Fat | Protein | Carbs | Fiber | Net Carbs |
| | | | | | | |
| | | | | | | |
| | | | | | | |
| Total: | | | | | | |
| **Dinner** | Calories | Fat | Protein | Carbs | Fiber | Net Carbs |
| | | | | | | |
| | | | | | | |
| | | | | | | |
| Total: | | | | | | |
| **Snacks** | Calories | Fat | Protein | Carbs | Fiber | Net Carbs |
| | | | | | | |
| | | | | | | |
| Total: | | | | | | |
| **Daily Total** | | | | | | |

**Ketosis:**   Y/N    Intermittent Fasting: From _____am/pm - To_____am/pm

# Day 61    Food Tracker    Date: _____
MON TUE WED THU FRI SAT SUN

| 🎯 Daily Target | | | | | | |
|---|---|---|---|---|---|---|
| **Breakfast** | Calories | Fat | Protein | Carbs | Fiber | Net Carbs |
| | | | | | | |
| | | | | | | |
| | | | | | | |
| | | | | | | |
| Total: | | | | | | |
| **Lunch** | Calories | Fat | Protein | Carbs | Fiber | Net Carbs |
| | | | | | | |
| | | | | | | |
| | | | | | | |
| | | | | | | |
| Total: | | | | | | |
| **Dinner** | Calories | Fat | Protein | Carbs | Fiber | Net Carbs |
| | | | | | | |
| | | | | | | |
| | | | | | | |
| | | | | | | |
| Total: | | | | | | |
| **Snacks** | Calories | Fat | Protein | Carbs | Fiber | Net Carbs |
| | | | | | | |
| | | | | | | |
| | | | | | | |
| Total: | | | | | | |
| **Daily Total** | | | | | | |

**Ketosis:**   Y/N      Intermittent Fasting: From _____am/pm - To_____am/pm

# Day 62    Food Tracker

| ⊕ Daily Target | | | | | | |
|---|---|---|---|---|---|---|
| **Breakfast** | Calories | Fat | Protein | Carbs | Fiber | Net Carbs |
| | | | | | | |
| | | | | | | |
| | | | | | | |
| | | | | | | |
| Total: | | | | | | |
| **Lunch** | Calories | Fat | Protein | Carbs | Fiber | Net Carbs |
| | | | | | | |
| | | | | | | |
| | | | | | | |
| | | | | | | |
| Total: | | | | | | |
| **Dinner** | Calories | Fat | Protein | Carbs | Fiber | Net Carbs |
| | | | | | | |
| | | | | | | |
| | | | | | | |
| | | | | | | |
| Total: | | | | | | |
| **Snacks** | Calories | Fat | Protein | Carbs | Fiber | Net Carbs |
| | | | | | | |
| | | | | | | |
| | | | | | | |
| Total: | | | | | | |
| **Daily Total** | | | | | | |

**Ketosis:**   Y/N    Intermittent Fasting: From _____am/pm - To_____am/pm

# Day 63　Food Tracker

Date: _____

| ⊕ Daily Target | | | | | | |
|---|---|---|---|---|---|---|

| **Breakfast** | Calories | Fat | Protein | Carbs | Fiber | Net Carbs |
|---|---|---|---|---|---|---|
| | | | | | | |
| | | | | | | |
| | | | | | | |
| Total: | | | | | | |

| **Lunch** | Calories | Fat | Protein | Carbs | Fiber | Net Carbs |
|---|---|---|---|---|---|---|
| | | | | | | |
| | | | | | | |
| | | | | | | |
| Total: | | | | | | |

| **Dinner** | Calories | Fat | Protein | Carbs | Fiber | Net Carbs |
|---|---|---|---|---|---|---|
| | | | | | | |
| | | | | | | |
| | | | | | | |
| Total: | | | | | | |

| **Snacks** | Calories | Fat | Protein | Carbs | Fiber | Net Carbs |
|---|---|---|---|---|---|---|
| | | | | | | |
| | | | | | | |
| Total: | | | | | | |

| **Daily Total** | | | | | | |
|---|---|---|---|---|---|---|

**Ketosis:**　Y/N　　Intermittent Fasting: From _____am/pm - To_____am/pm

# NOTES

# DAY 64 – WEIGHT

## Measurements

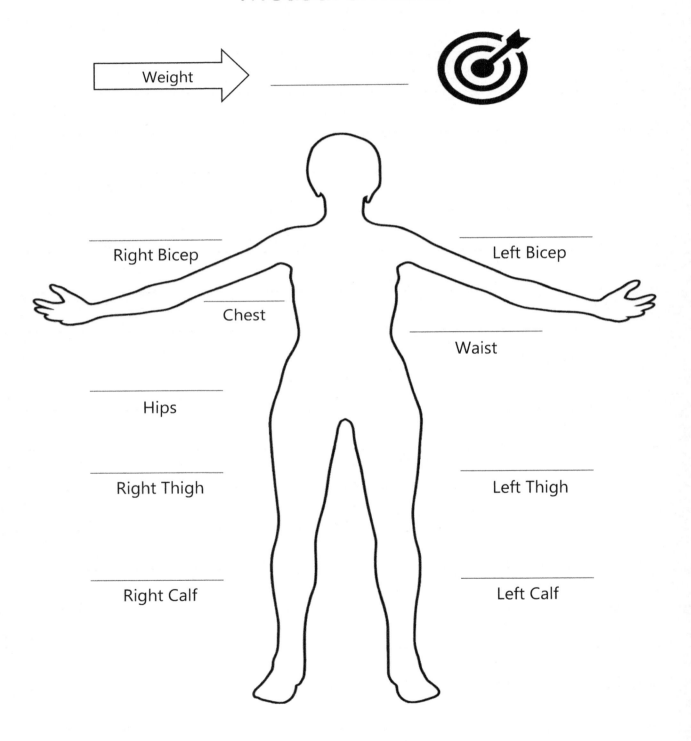

Weight ⟶ _____

Right Bicep

Left Bicep

Chest

Waist

Hips

Right Thigh

Left Thigh

Right Calf

Left Calf

# Questions To Ask Yourself

Am I happy with my results after the last 7 days?

_____

_____

_____

_____

What was my biggest win?

_____

_____

_____

What adjustments should I make?

_____

_____

_____

How does my body feel?

_____

_____

_____

# DAY 64 - 70

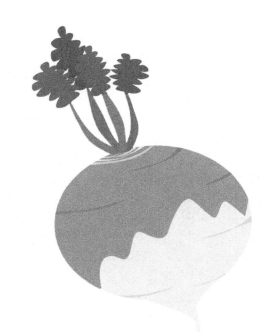

# Meal Planner

| | |
|---|---|
| Day 1 | Breakfast:<br>Lunch:<br>Dinner: |
| Day 2 | Breakfast:<br>Lunch:<br>Dinner: |
| Day 3 | Breakfast:<br>Lunch:<br>Dinner: |
| Day 4 | Breakfast:<br>Lunch:<br>Dinner: |
| Day 5 | Breakfast:<br>Lunch:<br>Dinner: |
| Day 6 | Breakfast:<br>Lunch:<br>Dinner: |
| Day 7 | Breakfast:<br>Lunch:<br>Dinner: |
| Snacks | |

# Exercise Tracker

Day 64 - 70

| Day 1 |
|---|
| |
| Cardio ◯ <br> Weights ◯ |

| Day 2 |
|---|
| |
| Cardio ◯ <br> Weights ◯ |

| Day 3 |
|---|
| |
| Cardio ◯ <br> Weights ◯ |

| Day 4 |
|---|
| |
| Cardio ◯ <br> Weights ◯ |

| Day 5 |
|---|
| |
| Cardio ◯ <br> Weights ◯ |

| Day 6 |
|---|
| |
| Cardio ◯ <br> Weights ◯ |

| Day 7 |
|---|
| |
| Cardio ◯ <br> Weights ◯ |

| Day | Calories Burned |
|---|---|
| 1 | |
| 2 | |
| 3 | |
| 4 | |
| 5 | |
| 6 | |
| 7 | |

# Day 64    Food Tracker    Date: _____

| ⊕ **Daily Target** | | | | | | |
|---|---|---|---|---|---|---|
| **Breakfast** | Calories | Fat | Protein | Carbs | Fiber | Net Carbs |
| | | | | | | |
| | | | | | | |
| | | | | | | |
| | | | | | | |
| Total: | | | | | | |
| **Lunch** | Calories | Fat | Protein | Carbs | Fiber | Net Carbs |
| | | | | | | |
| | | | | | | |
| | | | | | | |
| | | | | | | |
| Total: | | | | | | |
| **Dinner** | Calories | Fat | Protein | Carbs | Fiber | Net Carbs |
| | | | | | | |
| | | | | | | |
| | | | | | | |
| | | | | | | |
| Total: | | | | | | |
| **Snacks** | Calories | Fat | Protein | Carbs | Fiber | Net Carbs |
| | | | | | | |
| | | | | | | |
| | | | | | | |
| Total: | | | | | | |
| **Daily Total** | | | | | | |

**Ketosis:**    Y/N    Intermittent Fasting: From _____am/pm - To_____am/pm

# Day 65 Food Tracker

Date: _____

MON TUE WED THU FRI SAT SUN

| 🎯 Daily Target | | | | | | |
|---|---|---|---|---|---|---|
| **Breakfast** | Calories | Fat | Protein | Carbs | Fiber | Net Carbs |
| | | | | | | |
| | | | | | | |
| | | | | | | |
| | | | | | | |
| Total: | | | | | | |
| **Lunch** | Calories | Fat | Protein | Carbs | Fiber | Net Carbs |
| | | | | | | |
| | | | | | | |
| | | | | | | |
| | | | | | | |
| Total: | | | | | | |
| **Dinner** | Calories | Fat | Protein | Carbs | Fiber | Net Carbs |
| | | | | | | |
| | | | | | | |
| | | | | | | |
| | | | | | | |
| Total: | | | | | | |
| **Snacks** | Calories | Fat | Protein | Carbs | Fiber | Net Carbs |
| | | | | | | |
| | | | | | | |
| | | | | | | |
| Total: | | | | | | |
| **Daily Total** | | | | | | |

**Ketosis:**   Y/N    Intermittent Fasting: From _____am/pm - To_____am/pm

# Day 66    Food Tracker    Date: _____

| ⊕ Daily Target | | | | | | |
|---|---|---|---|---|---|---|
| **Breakfast** | Calories | Fat | Protein | Carbs | Fiber | Net Carbs |
| | | | | | | |
| | | | | | | |
| | | | | | | |
| | | | | | | |
| Total: | | | | | | |
| **Lunch** | Calories | Fat | Protein | Carbs | Fiber | Net Carbs |
| | | | | | | |
| | | | | | | |
| | | | | | | |
| | | | | | | |
| Total: | | | | | | |
| **Dinner** | Calories | Fat | Protein | Carbs | Fiber | Net Carbs |
| | | | | | | |
| | | | | | | |
| | | | | | | |
| | | | | | | |
| Total: | | | | | | |
| **Snacks** | Calories | Fat | Protein | Carbs | Fiber | Net Carbs |
| | | | | | | |
| | | | | | | |
| | | | | | | |
| Total: | | | | | | |
| **Daily Total** | | | | | | |

**Ketosis:**   Y/N    Intermittent Fasting: From _____am/pm  -  To_____am/pm

# Day 67    Food Tracker

| 🎯 Daily Target | | | | | | |
|---|---|---|---|---|---|---|
| **Breakfast** | Calories | Fat | Protein | Carbs | Fiber | Net Carbs |
| | | | | | | |
| | | | | | | |
| | | | | | | |
| | | | | | | |
| Total: | | | | | | |
| **Lunch** | Calories | Fat | Protein | Carbs | Fiber | Net Carbs |
| | | | | | | |
| | | | | | | |
| | | | | | | |
| | | | | | | |
| Total: | | | | | | |
| **Dinner** | Calories | Fat | Protein | Carbs | Fiber | Net Carbs |
| | | | | | | |
| | | | | | | |
| | | | | | | |
| | | | | | | |
| Total: | | | | | | |
| **Snacks** | Calories | Fat | Protein | Carbs | Fiber | Net Carbs |
| | | | | | | |
| | | | | | | |
| | | | | | | |
| Total: | | | | | | |
| **Daily Total** | | | | | | |

**Ketosis:**   Y/N    Intermittent Fasting: From _____am/pm - To_____am/pm

# Day 68　Food Tracker

| ⊕ Daily Target | | | | | | |
|---|---|---|---|---|---|---|
| **Breakfast** | Calories | Fat | Protein | Carbs | Fiber | Net Carbs |
| | | | | | | |
| | | | | | | |
| | | | | | | |
| Total: | | | | | | |
| **Lunch** | Calories | Fat | Protein | Carbs | Fiber | Net Carbs |
| | | | | | | |
| | | | | | | |
| | | | | | | |
| Total: | | | | | | |
| **Dinner** | Calories | Fat | Protein | Carbs | Fiber | Net Carbs |
| | | | | | | |
| | | | | | | |
| | | | | | | |
| | | | | | | |
| Total: | | | | | | |
| **Snacks** | Calories | Fat | Protein | Carbs | Fiber | Net Carbs |
| | | | | | | |
| | | | | | | |
| | | | | | | |
| Total: | | | | | | |
| **Daily Total** | | | | | | |

**Ketosis:**　Y/N　Intermittent Fasting: From _____am/pm - To_____am/pm

# Day 69    Food Tracker    Date: _____
MON TUE WED THU FRI SAT SUN

| ⊕ Daily Target | | | | | | |
|---|---|---|---|---|---|---|
| **Breakfast** | Calories | Fat | Protein | Carbs | Fiber | Net Carbs |
| | | | | | | |
| | | | | | | |
| | | | | | | |
| | | | | | | |
| Total: | | | | | | |
| **Lunch** | Calories | Fat | Protein | Carbs | Fiber | Net Carbs |
| | | | | | | |
| | | | | | | |
| | | | | | | |
| | | | | | | |
| Total: | | | | | | |
| **Dinner** | Calories | Fat | Protein | Carbs | Fiber | Net Carbs |
| | | | | | | |
| | | | | | | |
| | | | | | | |
| | | | | | | |
| Total: | | | | | | |
| **Snacks** | Calories | Fat | Protein | Carbs | Fiber | Net Carbs |
| | | | | | | |
| | | | | | | |
| | | | | | | |
| Total: | | | | | | |
| **Daily Total** | | | | | | |

**Ketosis:**   Y/N    Intermittent Fasting: From ____am/pm - To____am/pm

# Day 70    Food Tracker    Date: _____

| 🎯 Daily Target | | | | | | |
|---|---|---|---|---|---|---|
| **Breakfast** | Calories | Fat | Protein | Carbs | Fiber | Net Carbs |
| | | | | | | |
| | | | | | | |
| | | | | | | |
| | | | | | | |
| Total: | | | | | | |
| **Lunch** | Calories | Fat | Protein | Carbs | Fiber | Net Carbs |
| | | | | | | |
| | | | | | | |
| | | | | | | |
| | | | | | | |
| Total: | | | | | | |
| **Dinner** | Calories | Fat | Protein | Carbs | Fiber | Net Carbs |
| | | | | | | |
| | | | | | | |
| | | | | | | |
| | | | | | | |
| Total: | | | | | | |
| **Snacks** | Calories | Fat | Protein | Carbs | Fiber | Net Carbs |
| | | | | | | |
| | | | | | | |
| | | | | | | |
| Total: | | | | | | |
| **Daily Total** | | | | | | |

**Ketosis:** Y/N    Intermittent Fasting: From _____am/pm - To_____am/pm

# NOTES

# DAY 71 – WEIGHT

## Measurements

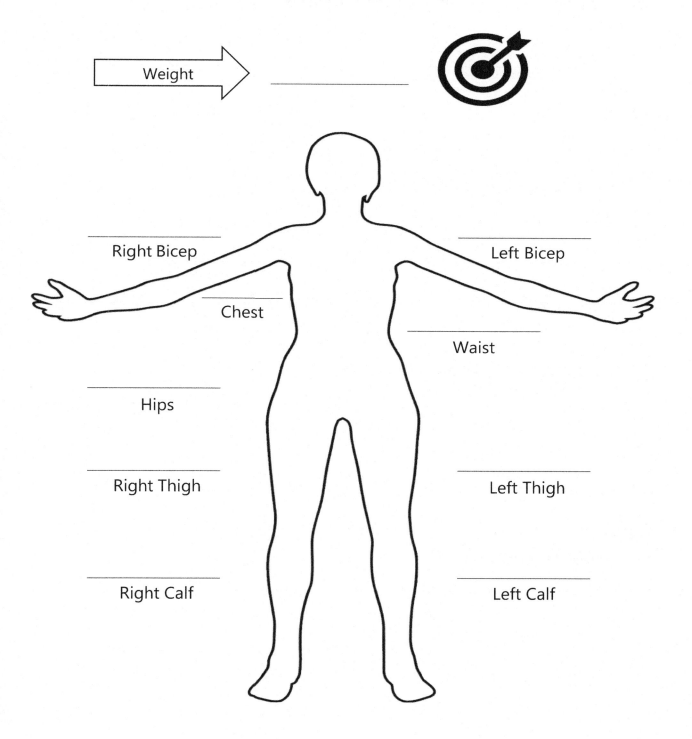

Weight

Right Bicep

Left Bicep

Chest

Waist

Hips

Right Thigh

Left Thigh

Right Calf

Left Calf

# Questions To Ask Yourself

Am I happy with my results after the last 7 days?

_____

_____

_____

_____

What was my biggest win?

_____

_____

_____

What adjustments should I make?

_____

_____

_____

How does my body feel?

_____

_____

_____

# DAY 71 - 77

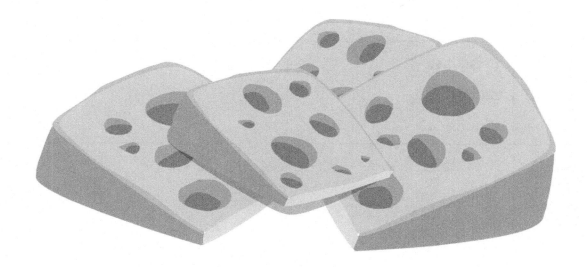

# Meal Planner

Day 71 - 77

| | |
|---|---|
| **Day 1** | Breakfast:<br><br>Lunch:<br><br>Dinner: |
| **Day 2** | Breakfast:<br><br>Lunch:<br><br>Dinner: |
| **Day 3** | Breakfast:<br><br>Lunch:<br><br>Dinner: |
| **Day 4** | Breakfast:<br><br>Lunch:<br><br>Dinner: |
| **Day 5** | Breakfast:<br><br>Lunch:<br><br>Dinner: |
| **Day 6** | Breakfast:<br><br>Lunch:<br><br>Dinner: |
| **Day 7** | Breakfast:<br><br>Lunch:<br><br>Dinner: |
| **Snacks** | |

# Exercise Tracker

| Day 1 | Day 2 | Day 3 |
|-------|-------|-------|
| | | |

| | | |
|---|---|---|
| Cardio ○<br>Weights ○ | Cardio ○<br>Weights ○ | Cardio ○<br>Weights ○ |

| Day 4 | Day 5 | Day 6 |
|-------|-------|-------|
| | | |

| | | |
|---|---|---|
| Cardio ○<br>Weights ○ | Cardio ○<br>Weights ○ | Cardio ○<br>Weights ○ |

| Day 7 |
|-------|
| |

Cardio ○
Weights ○

| Day | Calories Burned |
|-----|-----------------|
| 1 | |
| 2 | |
| 3 | |
| 4 | |
| 5 | |
| 6 | |
| 7 | |

# Day 71    Food Tracker    Date: _____

| 🎯 Daily Target | | | | | | |
|---|---|---|---|---|---|---|
| **Breakfast** | Calories | Fat | Protein | Carbs | Fiber | Net Carbs |
| | | | | | | |
| | | | | | | |
| | | | | | | |
| | | | | | | |
| Total: | | | | | | |
| **Lunch** | Calories | Fat | Protein | Carbs | Fiber | Net Carbs |
| | | | | | | |
| | | | | | | |
| | | | | | | |
| | | | | | | |
| Total: | | | | | | |
| **Dinner** | Calories | Fat | Protein | Carbs | Fiber | Net Carbs |
| | | | | | | |
| | | | | | | |
| | | | | | | |
| | | | | | | |
| | | | | | | |
| Total: | | | | | | |
| **Snacks** | Calories | Fat | Protein | Carbs | Fiber | Net Carbs |
| | | | | | | |
| | | | | | | |
| | | | | | | |
| Total: | | | | | | |
| **Daily Total** | | | | | | |

**Ketosis:**   Y/N    Intermittent Fasting: From _____am/pm - To_____am/pm

# Day 72    Food Tracker

Date: _____
MON TUE WED THU FRI SAT SUN

| 🎯 Daily Target | | | | | | |
|---|---|---|---|---|---|---|
| **Breakfast** | Calories | Fat | Protein | Carbs | Fiber | Net Carbs |
| | | | | | | |
| | | | | | | |
| | | | | | | |
| | | | | | | |
| Total: | | | | | | |
| **Lunch** | Calories | Fat | Protein | Carbs | Fiber | Net Carbs |
| | | | | | | |
| | | | | | | |
| | | | | | | |
| | | | | | | |
| Total: | | | | | | |
| **Dinner** | Calories | Fat | Protein | Carbs | Fiber | Net Carbs |
| | | | | | | |
| | | | | | | |
| | | | | | | |
| | | | | | | |
| Total: | | | | | | |
| **Snacks** | Calories | Fat | Protein | Carbs | Fiber | Net Carbs |
| | | | | | | |
| | | | | | | |
| | | | | | | |
| Total: | | | | | | |
| **Daily Total** | | | | | | |

**Ketosis:**   Y/N    Intermittent Fasting: From _____am/pm - To_____am/pm

# Day 73    Food Tracker     Date: _____

| 🎯 **Daily Target** | | | | | | |
|---|---|---|---|---|---|---|

| **Breakfast** | Calories | Fat | Protein | Carbs | Fiber | Net Carbs |
|---|---|---|---|---|---|---|
| | | | | | | |
| | | | | | | |
| | | | | | | |
| | | | | | | |
| Total: | | | | | | |

| **Lunch** | Calories | Fat | Protein | Carbs | Fiber | Net Carbs |
|---|---|---|---|---|---|---|
| | | | | | | |
| | | | | | | |
| | | | | | | |
| | | | | | | |
| Total: | | | | | | |

| **Dinner** | Calories | Fat | Protein | Carbs | Fiber | Net Carbs |
|---|---|---|---|---|---|---|
| | | | | | | |
| | | | | | | |
| | | | | | | |
| | | | | | | |
| Total: | | | | | | |

| **Snacks** | Calories | Fat | Protein | Carbs | Fiber | Net Carbs |
|---|---|---|---|---|---|---|
| | | | | | | |
| | | | | | | |
| | | | | | | |
| Total: | | | | | | |

| **Daily Total** | | | | | | |
|---|---|---|---|---|---|---|

**Ketosis:**   Y/N     Intermittent Fasting: From _____am/pm - To_____am/pm

# Day 74     Food Tracker     Date: _____

| ⊕ Daily Target | | | | | | |
|---|---|---|---|---|---|---|
| **Breakfast** | Calories | Fat | Protein | Carbs | Fiber | Net Carbs |
| | | | | | | |
| | | | | | | |
| | | | | | | |
| Total: | | | | | | |
| **Lunch** | Calories | Fat | Protein | Carbs | Fiber | Net Carbs |
| | | | | | | |
| | | | | | | |
| | | | | | | |
| Total: | | | | | | |
| **Dinner** | Calories | Fat | Protein | Carbs | Fiber | Net Carbs |
| | | | | | | |
| | | | | | | |
| | | | | | | |
| | | | | | | |
| Total: | | | | | | |
| **Snacks** | Calories | Fat | Protein | Carbs | Fiber | Net Carbs |
| | | | | | | |
| | | | | | | |
| | | | | | | |
| Total: | | | | | | |
| **Daily Total** | | | | | | |

**Ketosis:**   Y/N     Intermittent Fasting: From _____am/pm  -  To_____am/pm

# Day 75     Food Tracker     Date: _____
MON TUE WED THU FRI SAT SUN

| ⊕ Daily Target | | | | | | |
|---|---|---|---|---|---|---|

| Breakfast | Calories | Fat | Protein | Carbs | Fiber | Net Carbs |
|---|---|---|---|---|---|---|
|  |  |  |  |  |  |  |
|  |  |  |  |  |  |  |
|  |  |  |  |  |  |  |
|  |  |  |  |  |  |  |
| Total: |  |  |  |  |  |  |

| Lunch | Calories | Fat | Protein | Carbs | Fiber | Net Carbs |
|---|---|---|---|---|---|---|
|  |  |  |  |  |  |  |
|  |  |  |  |  |  |  |
|  |  |  |  |  |  |  |
|  |  |  |  |  |  |  |
| Total: |  |  |  |  |  |  |

| Dinner | Calories | Fat | Protein | Carbs | Fiber | Net Carbs |
|---|---|---|---|---|---|---|
|  |  |  |  |  |  |  |
|  |  |  |  |  |  |  |
|  |  |  |  |  |  |  |
|  |  |  |  |  |  |  |
| Total: |  |  |  |  |  |  |

| Snacks | Calories | Fat | Protein | Carbs | Fiber | Net Carbs |
|---|---|---|---|---|---|---|
|  |  |  |  |  |  |  |
|  |  |  |  |  |  |  |
|  |  |  |  |  |  |  |
| Total: |  |  |  |  |  |  |

| Daily Total | | | | | | |
|---|---|---|---|---|---|---|

**Ketosis:**   Y/N     Intermittent Fasting: From _____am/pm  -  To_____am/pm

# Day 76    Food Tracker

| 🎯 Daily Target | | | | | | |
|---|---|---|---|---|---|---|
| **Breakfast** | Calories | Fat | Protein | Carbs | Fiber | Net Carbs |
| | | | | | | |
| | | | | | | |
| | | | | | | |
| Total: | | | | | | |
| **Lunch** | Calories | Fat | Protein | Carbs | Fiber | Net Carbs |
| | | | | | | |
| | | | | | | |
| | | | | | | |
| Total: | | | | | | |
| **Dinner** | Calories | Fat | Protein | Carbs | Fiber | Net Carbs |
| | | | | | | |
| | | | | | | |
| | | | | | | |
| | | | | | | |
| Total: | | | | | | |
| **Snacks** | Calories | Fat | Protein | Carbs | Fiber | Net Carbs |
| | | | | | | |
| | | | | | | |
| | | | | | | |
| Total: | | | | | | |
| **Daily Total** | | | | | | |

**Ketosis:**   Y/N    Intermittent Fasting: From _____am/pm - To_____am/pm

# Day 77    Food Tracker    Date: _____

| 🎯 Daily Target | | | | | | |
|---|---|---|---|---|---|---|

| Breakfast | Calories | Fat | Protein | Carbs | Fiber | Net Carbs |
|---|---|---|---|---|---|---|
| | | | | | | |
| | | | | | | |
| | | | | | | |
| | | | | | | |
| Total: | | | | | | |

| Lunch | Calories | Fat | Protein | Carbs | Fiber | Net Carbs |
|---|---|---|---|---|---|---|
| | | | | | | |
| | | | | | | |
| | | | | | | |
| | | | | | | |
| Total: | | | | | | |

| Dinner | Calories | Fat | Protein | Carbs | Fiber | Net Carbs |
|---|---|---|---|---|---|---|
| | | | | | | |
| | | | | | | |
| | | | | | | |
| | | | | | | |
| Total: | | | | | | |

| Snacks | Calories | Fat | Protein | Carbs | Fiber | Net Carbs |
|---|---|---|---|---|---|---|
| | | | | | | |
| | | | | | | |
| | | | | | | |
| Total: | | | | | | |

| Daily Total | | | | | | |
|---|---|---|---|---|---|---|

**Ketosis:**    Y/N    Intermittent Fasting: From _____am/pm - To_____am/pm

# NOTES

# DAY 78 – WEIGHT

## Measurements

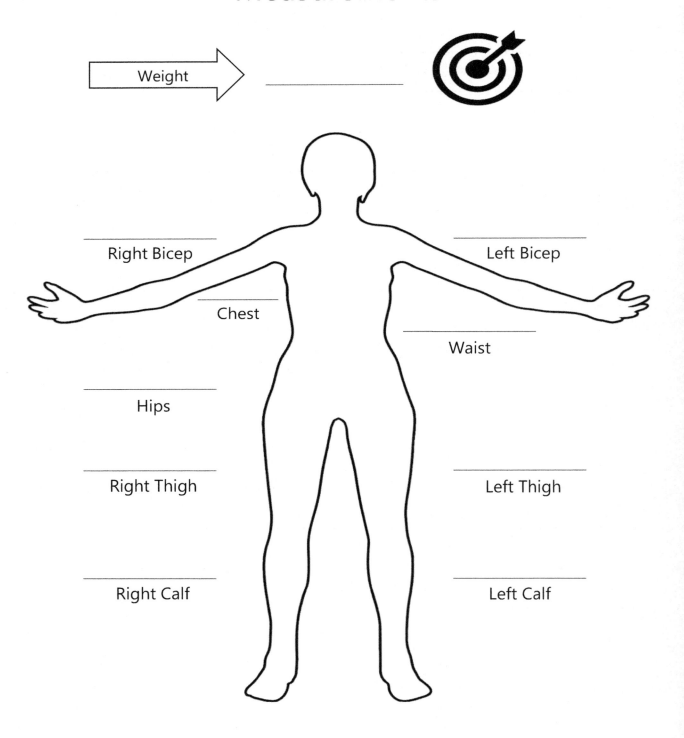

Weight →

Right Bicep

Left Bicep

Chest

Waist

Hips

Right Thigh

Left Thigh

Right Calf

Left Calf

# Questions To Ask Yourself

Am I happy with my results after the last 7 days?

_____

_____

_____

_____

What was my biggest win?

_____

_____

_____

_____

What adjustments should I make?

_____

_____

_____

_____

How does my body feel?

_____

_____

_____

_____

# DAY 78 - 84

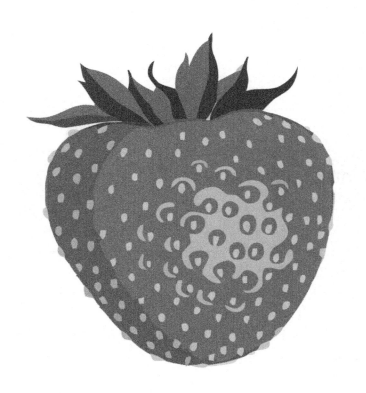

# Meal Planner

Day 78 - 84

| | |
|---|---|
| Day 1 | Breakfast:<br><br>Lunch:<br><br>Dinner: |
| Day 2 | Breakfast:<br><br>Lunch:<br><br>Dinner: |
| Day 3 | Breakfast:<br><br>Lunch:<br><br>Dinner: |
| Day 4 | Breakfast:<br><br>Lunch:<br><br>Dinner: |
| Day 5 | Breakfast:<br><br>Lunch:<br><br>Dinner: |
| Day 6 | Breakfast:<br><br>Lunch:<br><br>Dinner: |
| Day 7 | Breakfast:<br><br>Lunch:<br><br>Dinner: |
| Snacks | |

# Exercise Tracker

| Day 1 |
|---|

Cardio ⭕
Weights ⭕

| Day 2 |
|---|

Cardio ⭕
Weights ⭕

| Day 3 |
|---|

Cardio ⭕
Weights ⭕

| Day 4 |
|---|

Cardio ⭕
Weights ⭕

| Day 5 |
|---|

Cardio ⭕
Weights ⭕

| Day 6 |
|---|

Cardio ⭕
Weights ⭕

| Day 7 |
|---|

Cardio ⭕
Weights ⭕

| Day | Calories Burned |
|---|---|
| 1 | |
| 2 | |
| 3 | |
| 4 | |
| 5 | |
| 6 | |
| 7 | |

# Day 78    Food Tracker    Date: _____

| 🎯 Daily Target | | | | | | |
|---|---|---|---|---|---|---|
| **Breakfast** | Calories | Fat | Protein | Carbs | Fiber | Net Carbs |
| | | | | | | |
| | | | | | | |
| | | | | | | |
| Total: | | | | | | |
| **Lunch** | Calories | Fat | Protein | Carbs | Fiber | Net Carbs |
| | | | | | | |
| | | | | | | |
| | | | | | | |
| | | | | | | |
| Total: | | | | | | |
| **Dinner** | Calories | Fat | Protein | Carbs | Fiber | Net Carbs |
| | | | | | | |
| | | | | | | |
| | | | | | | |
| | | | | | | |
| Total: | | | | | | |
| **Snacks** | Calories | Fat | Protein | Carbs | Fiber | Net Carbs |
| | | | | | | |
| | | | | | | |
| | | | | | | |
| Total: | | | | | | |
| **Daily Total** | | | | | | |

**Ketosis:**   Y/N    Intermittent Fasting: From _____am/pm - To_____am/pm

# Day 79    Food Tracker    Date: _____
MON TUE WED THU FRI SAT SUN

| ⊕ **Daily Target** | | | | | | |
|---|---|---|---|---|---|---|
| **Breakfast** | Calories | Fat | Protein | Carbs | Fiber | Net Carbs |
| | | | | | | |
| | | | | | | |
| | | | | | | |
| | | | | | | |
| Total: | | | | | | |
| **Lunch** | Calories | Fat | Protein | Carbs | Fiber | Net Carbs |
| | | | | | | |
| | | | | | | |
| | | | | | | |
| | | | | | | |
| Total: | | | | | | |
| **Dinner** | Calories | Fat | Protein | Carbs | Fiber | Net Carbs |
| | | | | | | |
| | | | | | | |
| | | | | | | |
| | | | | | | |
| Total: | | | | | | |
| **Snacks** | Calories | Fat | Protein | Carbs | Fiber | Net Carbs |
| | | | | | | |
| | | | | | | |
| | | | | | | |
| Total: | | | | | | |
| **Daily Total** | | | | | | |

**Ketosis:**   Y/N      Intermittent Fasting: From _____am/pm - To_____am/pm

# Day 80    Food Tracker    Date: _____

MON TUE WED THU FRI SAT SUN

| ⊕ Daily Target | | | | | | |
|---|---|---|---|---|---|---|
| **Breakfast** | Calories | Fat | Protein | Carbs | Fiber | Net Carbs |
| | | | | | | |
| | | | | | | |
| | | | | | | |
| | | | | | | |
| Total: | | | | | | |
| **Lunch** | Calories | Fat | Protein | Carbs | Fiber | Net Carbs |
| | | | | | | |
| | | | | | | |
| | | | | | | |
| | | | | | | |
| Total: | | | | | | |
| **Dinner** | Calories | Fat | Protein | Carbs | Fiber | Net Carbs |
| | | | | | | |
| | | | | | | |
| | | | | | | |
| | | | | | | |
| Total: | | | | | | |
| **Snacks** | Calories | Fat | Protein | Carbs | Fiber | Net Carbs |
| | | | | | | |
| | | | | | | |
| | | | | | | |
| Total: | | | | | | |
| **Daily Total** | | | | | | |

**Ketosis:**   Y/N      Intermittent Fasting: From _____am/pm  -  To_____am/pm

# Day 81    Food Tracker

Date: _____

MON TUE WED THU FRI SAT SUN

| 🎯 Daily Target | | | | | | |
|---|---|---|---|---|---|---|
| **Breakfast** | Calories | Fat | Protein | Carbs | Fiber | Net Carbs |
| | | | | | | |
| | | | | | | |
| | | | | | | |
| | | | | | | |
| Total: | | | | | | |
| **Lunch** | Calories | Fat | Protein | Carbs | Fiber | Net Carbs |
| | | | | | | |
| | | | | | | |
| | | | | | | |
| | | | | | | |
| Total: | | | | | | |
| **Dinner** | Calories | Fat | Protein | Carbs | Fiber | Net Carbs |
| | | | | | | |
| | | | | | | |
| | | | | | | |
| | | | | | | |
| Total: | | | | | | |
| **Snacks** | Calories | Fat | Protein | Carbs | Fiber | Net Carbs |
| | | | | | | |
| | | | | | | |
| | | | | | | |
| Total: | | | | | | |
| **Daily Total** | | | | | | |

**Ketosis:**    Y/N    Intermittent Fasting: From _____am/pm  -  To_____am/pm

# Day 82     Food Tracker     Date: _____

| 🎯 Daily Target | | | | | | |
|---|---|---|---|---|---|---|
| **Breakfast** | Calories | Fat | Protein | Carbs | Fiber | Net Carbs |
| | | | | | | |
| | | | | | | |
| | | | | | | |
| Total: | | | | | | |
| **Lunch** | Calories | Fat | Protein | Carbs | Fiber | Net Carbs |
| | | | | | | |
| | | | | | | |
| | | | | | | |
| | | | | | | |
| Total: | | | | | | |
| **Dinner** | Calories | Fat | Protein | Carbs | Fiber | Net Carbs |
| | | | | | | |
| | | | | | | |
| | | | | | | |
| | | | | | | |
| Total: | | | | | | |
| **Snacks** | Calories | Fat | Protein | Carbs | Fiber | Net Carbs |
| | | | | | | |
| | | | | | | |
| | | | | | | |
| Total: | | | | | | |
| **Daily Total** | | | | | | |

**Ketosis:**   Y/N      Intermittent Fasting: From _____am/pm  - To_____am/pm

# Day 83    Food Tracker    Date: _____

| ⊕ **Daily Target** | | | | | | |
|---|---|---|---|---|---|---|
| **Breakfast** | Calories | Fat | Protein | Carbs | Fiber | Net Carbs |
| | | | | | | |
| | | | | | | |
| | | | | | | |
| | | | | | | |
| Total: | | | | | | |
| **Lunch** | Calories | Fat | Protein | Carbs | Fiber | Net Carbs |
| | | | | | | |
| | | | | | | |
| | | | | | | |
| | | | | | | |
| Total: | | | | | | |
| **Dinner** | Calories | Fat | Protein | Carbs | Fiber | Net Carbs |
| | | | | | | |
| | | | | | | |
| | | | | | | |
| | | | | | | |
| Total: | | | | | | |
| **Snacks** | Calories | Fat | Protein | Carbs | Fiber | Net Carbs |
| | | | | | | |
| | | | | | | |
| | | | | | | |
| Total: | | | | | | |
| **Daily Total** | | | | | | |

**Ketosis:** Y/N    Intermittent Fasting: From _____am/pm - To_____am/pm

# Day 84  Food Tracker

Date: _____

| ⊕ Daily Target | | | | | | |
|---|---|---|---|---|---|---|
| **Breakfast** | Calories | Fat | Protein | Carbs | Fiber | Net Carbs |
| | | | | | | |
| | | | | | | |
| | | | | | | |
| Total: | | | | | | |
| **Lunch** | Calories | Fat | Protein | Carbs | Fiber | Net Carbs |
| | | | | | | |
| | | | | | | |
| | | | | | | |
| Total: | | | | | | |
| **Dinner** | Calories | Fat | Protein | Carbs | Fiber | Net Carbs |
| | | | | | | |
| | | | | | | |
| | | | | | | |
| Total: | | | | | | |
| **Snacks** | Calories | Fat | Protein | Carbs | Fiber | Net Carbs |
| | | | | | | |
| | | | | | | |
| | | | | | | |
| Total: | | | | | | |
| **Daily Total** | | | | | | |

**Ketosis:**  Y/N     Intermittent Fasting: From _____am/pm - To_____am/pm

# NOTES

# DAY 85 – WEIGHT

## Measurements

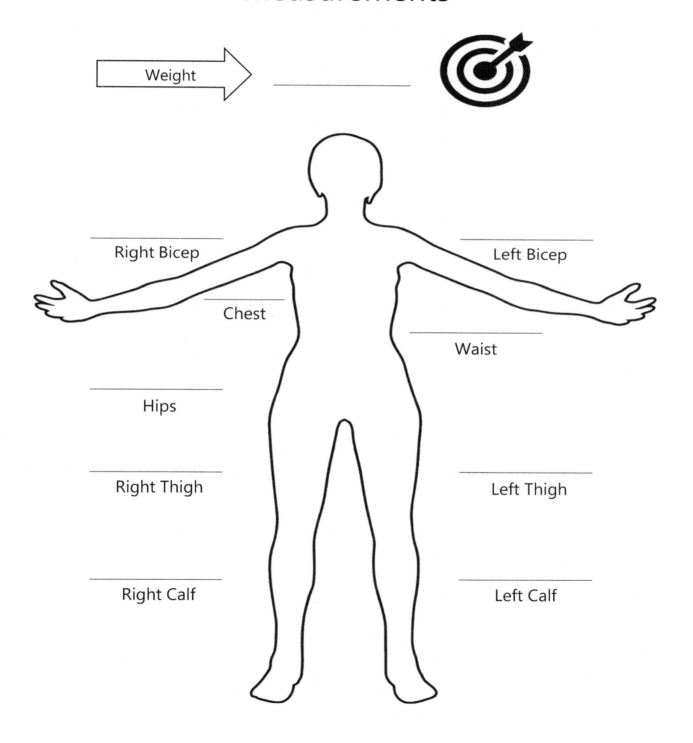

Weight ⟶ _____

Right Bicep

Left Bicep

Chest

Waist

Hips

Right Thigh

Left Thigh

Right Calf

Left Calf

# Questions To Ask Yourself

Am I happy with my results after the last 7 days?

_____

_____

_____

_____

What was my biggest win?

_____

_____

_____

What adjustments should I make?

_____

_____

_____

How does my body feel?

_____

_____

_____

_____

# DAY 85 - 90

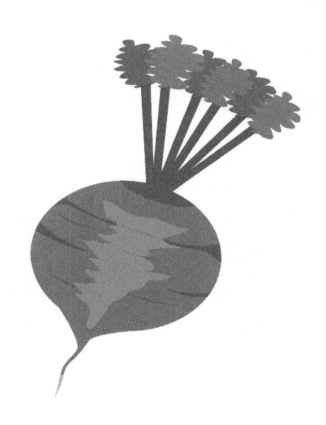

# Meal Planner

| | |
|---|---|
| Day 1 | Breakfast:<br>Lunch:<br>Dinner: |
| Day 2 | Breakfast:<br>Lunch:<br>Dinner: |
| Day 3 | Breakfast:<br>Lunch:<br>Dinner: |
| Day 4 | Breakfast:<br>Lunch:<br>Dinner: |
| Day 5 | Breakfast:<br>Lunch:<br>Dinner: |
| Day 6 | Breakfast:<br>Lunch:<br>Dinner: |
| Day 7 | Breakfast:<br>Lunch:<br>Dinner: |
| Snacks | |

# Exercise Tracker

Day 85 - 90

| Day 1 | Day 2 | Day 3 |
|---|---|---|
| | | |
| Cardio ◯<br>Weights ◯ | Cardio ◯<br>Weights ◯ | Cardio ◯<br>Weights ◯ |

| Day 4 | Day 5 | Day 6 |
|---|---|---|
| | | |
| Cardio ◯<br>Weights ◯ | Cardio ◯<br>Weights ◯ | Cardio ◯<br>Weights ◯ |

| Day 7 | Day | Calories Burned |
|---|---|---|
| | 1 | |
| | 2 | |
| | 3 | |
| | 4 | |
| | 5 | |
| Cardio ◯ | 6 | |
| Weights ◯ | 7 | |

# Day 85　Food Tracker

Date: _____
MON TUE WED THU FRI SAT SUN

| 🎯 **Daily Target** | | | | | | |
|---|---|---|---|---|---|---|
| **Breakfast** | Calories | Fat | Protein | Carbs | Fiber | Net Carbs |
| | | | | | | |
| | | | | | | |
| | | | | | | |
| | | | | | | |
| Total: | | | | | | |
| **Lunch** | Calories | Fat | Protein | Carbs | Fiber | Net Carbs |
| | | | | | | |
| | | | | | | |
| | | | | | | |
| | | | | | | |
| Total: | | | | | | |
| **Dinner** | Calories | Fat | Protein | Carbs | Fiber | Net Carbs |
| | | | | | | |
| | | | | | | |
| | | | | | | |
| | | | | | | |
| Total: | | | | | | |
| **Snacks** | Calories | Fat | Protein | Carbs | Fiber | Net Carbs |
| | | | | | | |
| | | | | | | |
| | | | | | | |
| Total: | | | | | | |
| **Daily Total** | | | | | | |

**Ketosis:** Y/N　Intermittent Fasting: From _____am/pm - To_____am/pm

# Day 86    Food Tracker

Date: _____

MON TUE WED THU FRI SAT SUN

| 🎯 Daily Target | | | | | | |
|---|---|---|---|---|---|---|
| **Breakfast** | Calories | Fat | Protein | Carbs | Fiber | Net Carbs |
| | | | | | | |
| | | | | | | |
| | | | | | | |
| | | | | | | |
| Total: | | | | | | |
| **Lunch** | Calories | Fat | Protein | Carbs | Fiber | Net Carbs |
| | | | | | | |
| | | | | | | |
| | | | | | | |
| | | | | | | |
| Total: | | | | | | |
| **Dinner** | Calories | Fat | Protein | Carbs | Fiber | Net Carbs |
| | | | | | | |
| | | | | | | |
| | | | | | | |
| | | | | | | |
| Total: | | | | | | |
| **Snacks** | Calories | Fat | Protein | Carbs | Fiber | Net Carbs |
| | | | | | | |
| | | | | | | |
| | | | | | | |
| Total: | | | | | | |
| **Daily Total** | | | | | | |

**Ketosis:**   Y/N    Intermittent Fasting: From _____am/pm  -  To_____am/pm

# Day 87    Food Tracker

Date: _____

MON TUE WED THU FRI SAT SUN

| 🎯 Daily Target | | | | | | |
|---|---|---|---|---|---|---|
| **Breakfast** | Calories | Fat | Protein | Carbs | Fiber | Net Carbs |
| | | | | | | |
| | | | | | | |
| | | | | | | |
| | | | | | | |
| Total: | | | | | | |
| **Lunch** | Calories | Fat | Protein | Carbs | Fiber | Net Carbs |
| | | | | | | |
| | | | | | | |
| | | | | | | |
| | | | | | | |
| Total: | | | | | | |
| **Dinner** | Calories | Fat | Protein | Carbs | Fiber | Net Carbs |
| | | | | | | |
| | | | | | | |
| | | | | | | |
| | | | | | | |
| | | | | | | |
| Total: | | | | | | |
| **Snacks** | Calories | Fat | Protein | Carbs | Fiber | Net Carbs |
| | | | | | | |
| | | | | | | |
| | | | | | | |
| Total: | | | | | | |
| **Daily Total** | | | | | | |

**Ketosis:**   Y/N    Intermittent Fasting: From _____am/pm - To_____am/pm

# Day 88    Food Tracker

Date: _____

MON TUE WED THU FRI SAT SUN

| ⊕ **Daily Target** | | | | | | |
|---|---|---|---|---|---|---|
| **Breakfast** | Calories | Fat | Protein | Carbs | Fiber | Net Carbs |
| | | | | | | |
| | | | | | | |
| | | | | | | |
| Total: | | | | | | |
| **Lunch** | Calories | Fat | Protein | Carbs | Fiber | Net Carbs |
| | | | | | | |
| | | | | | | |
| | | | | | | |
| Total: | | | | | | |
| **Dinner** | Calories | Fat | Protein | Carbs | Fiber | Net Carbs |
| | | | | | | |
| | | | | | | |
| | | | | | | |
| | | | | | | |
| Total: | | | | | | |
| **Snacks** | Calories | Fat | Protein | Carbs | Fiber | Net Carbs |
| | | | | | | |
| | | | | | | |
| | | | | | | |
| Total: | | | | | | |
| **Daily Total** | | | | | | |

**Ketosis:**   Y/N    Intermittent Fasting: From _____am/pm - To_____am/pm

# Day 89    Food Tracker

Date: _____

MON TUE WED THU FRI SAT SUN

| ⊕ Daily Target | | | | | | |
|---|---|---|---|---|---|---|
| **Breakfast** | Calories | Fat | Protein | Carbs | Fiber | Net Carbs |
| | | | | | | |
| | | | | | | |
| | | | | | | |
| | | | | | | |
| Total: | | | | | | |
| **Lunch** | Calories | Fat | Protein | Carbs | Fiber | Net Carbs |
| | | | | | | |
| | | | | | | |
| | | | | | | |
| | | | | | | |
| Total: | | | | | | |
| **Dinner** | Calories | Fat | Protein | Carbs | Fiber | Net Carbs |
| | | | | | | |
| | | | | | | |
| | | | | | | |
| | | | | | | |
| Total: | | | | | | |
| **Snacks** | Calories | Fat | Protein | Carbs | Fiber | Net Carbs |
| | | | | | | |
| | | | | | | |
| | | | | | | |
| | | | | | | |
| Total: | | | | | | |
| **Daily Total** | | | | | | |

**Ketosis:**   Y/N    Intermittent Fasting: From _____am/pm - To_____am/pm

# Day 90    Food Tracker    Date: _____

| 🎯 Daily Target | | | | | | |
|---|---|---|---|---|---|---|
| **Breakfast** | Calories | Fat | Protein | Carbs | Fiber | Net Carbs |
| | | | | | | |
| | | | | | | |
| | | | | | | |
| | | | | | | |
| Total: | | | | | | |
| **Lunch** | Calories | Fat | Protein | Carbs | Fiber | Net Carbs |
| | | | | | | |
| | | | | | | |
| | | | | | | |
| | | | | | | |
| Total: | | | | | | |
| **Dinner** | Calories | Fat | Protein | Carbs | Fiber | Net Carbs |
| | | | | | | |
| | | | | | | |
| | | | | | | |
| | | | | | | |
| Total: | | | | | | |
| **Snacks** | Calories | Fat | Protein | Carbs | Fiber | Net Carbs |
| | | | | | | |
| | | | | | | |
| | | | | | | |
| Total: | | | | | | |
| **Daily Total** | | | | | | |

**Ketosis:**   Y/N     Intermittent Fasting: From _____am/pm  -  To_____am/pm

# NOTES

# DAY 90 – ENDING WEIGHT

## Measurements

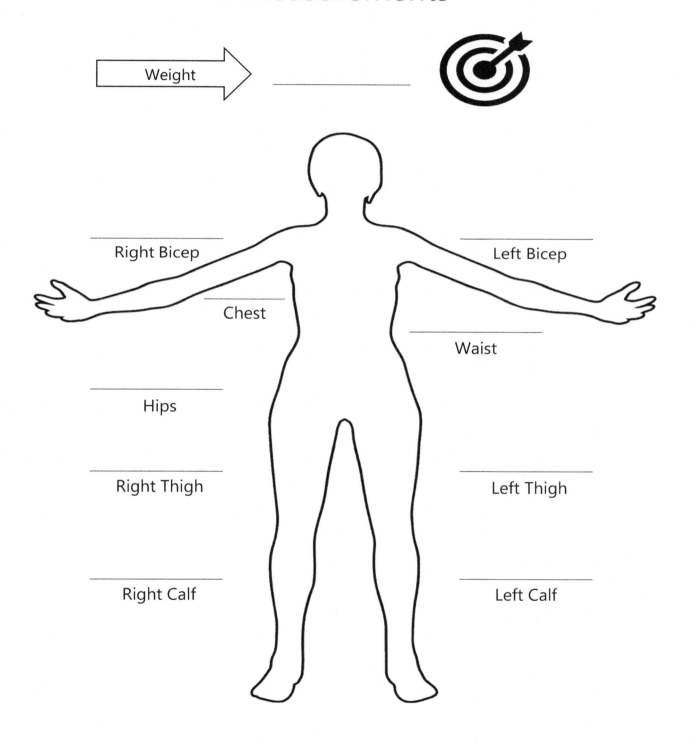

Weight ⟶ _____

Right Bicep

Left Bicep

Chest

Waist

Hips

Right Thigh

Left Thigh

Right Calf

Left Calf

# Questions To Ask Yourself

Am I happy with my results after the last 90 days?

_____

_____

_____

_____

What was my biggest win?

_____

_____

_____

What adjustments should I make?

_____

_____

_____

How does my body feel?

_____

_____

_____

_____

# NOTES

# NOTES

# NOTES

# NOTES

# NOTES

Printed in Great Britain
by Amazon

42315345R00099